HOW TO KEEP YOUR BRAIN YOUNG

H. NORMAN WRIGHT

H. Norman Wright (signature)

HARVEST HOUSE PUBLISHERS
EUGENE, OREGON

Cover design by Kyler Dougherty

Interior design by Angie Renich / Wildwood Digital Publishing

Cover photo ©serkorkin/gettyimages

For bulk, special sales, or ministry purchases, please call 1-800-547-8979. Email: Customerservice@hhpbooks.com

How to Keep Your Brain Young

Copyright © 2020 by H. Norman Wright
Published by Harvest House Publishers
Eugene, Oregon 97408
www.harvesthousepublishers.com

ISBN 978-0-7369-8055-5 (pbk.)
ISBN 978-0-7369-8056-2 (eBook)

Library of Congress Control Number: 2020946053

Contents

*I praise you, for I am fearfully
and wonderfully made.
Wonderful are your works;
my soul knows it very well.*

Psalm 139:14 ESV

PART ONE

CHAPTER 1

How's Your Brain?

Imagine this. You go to your doctor for a yearly checkup. You wait for a while, thumbing through some magazines or checking your smartphone. Finally, a nurse or technician comes out and leads you into a small, sterile examining room, which is quite cold and unfriendly, and there you wait some more. You hear footsteps coming down the hall, but then they disappear.

Finally—yes, finally—the door opens, and your doctor or PA appears. Since this is a yearly exam, the doctor wants to be thorough, so the questions begin. You're ready with a list of symptoms to discuss, from the big problems to the small pains that come and go from day to day. You want to know what those aches and pains mean...or do you? What if it could be cancer? What if it could be inoperable? What if it could be the beginning of an incapacitating disease? Because your third cousin had that illness at 35, and Aunt Janice and your mother died too early...

But the doctor's first question is not what you expect. He looks at your chest and then looks at you and says, "How's your brain?"

Silence.

"How's my brain? What kind of question is *that*?"

I've never actually been asked that question, and you probably haven't either. But we should ask ourselves this question, for the brain is the foundation of much of our lives.

It's a mystery. It only weighs three pounds, regardless of your weight. Without this organ, your heart wouldn't beat, your lungs wouldn't breathe, and your limbs would be immobilized.

This unique mass directs what you do. Your brain is a series of complex systems that sustain life. It was working before you were born. Your brain is constantly on call. It tells your heart what to do continually. If you want air, it directs your lungs to breathe. Your brain has the consistency of gelatin. It's cushioned from everyday jolts and bumps by cerebrospinal fluid inside your skull. A violent blow to your head and neck or upper body can cause your brain to slide back and forth forcefully against the walls of your skull. And over 90 percent of what we know about the brain has been discovered in the last ten years. It's involved in all you experience in life.[1]

We were created in such a marvelous way, especially our brain. Perhaps this passage from Scripture describes it best: "I praise you because I am fearfully and wonderfully made; your works are wonderful, I know that full well" (Psalm 139:14).

Build Your Muscles

This is the era of building our bodies (at least for some of us). I've had friends spend two hours a day at the gym trying to add some bulk onto their body. They grunt, sweat, and keep at it, hoping their muscles will reflect the results of aging. One day I asked one of them what his workout routine was as well as his purpose. He said, "I go through all of this to keep my body in shape. I don't want my muscles to become flabby. I want to increase their strength. I want to look better as well (that was questionable). When I work out, I'm more alert and sharper at my work. I feel energized. I want muscle strength. And I want others to notice me more, you know..."

I replied with, "So are you working on every muscle?"

He answered, "I think I've identified every muscle, and I have a program for each one."

I then asked, "What about your brain? What's your workout plan for your brain?"

Silence—more silence. He looked at me as though I had lost it and said, "What are you talking about? This is a gym—you know—build muscles. The body, not the mind."

He walked away shaking his head like I'd lost my mind! But it's true.

The facts are simple: Your brain is like a muscle, and it needs exercise. Its substance may be different, but plain and simple, like any muscle, it needs exercise to stay healthy. But how do you accomplish this? From this point on, think about strengthening your brain. Your brain needs a workout, and you may be surprised to learn that the best way for this to occur is information! Yes, plain old information. It's any kind of information which activates the neurons (these will be discussed later) in your head. But at the same time, we can feed our body. We need many kinds of good, solid information, and this includes learning about neurons (yes, we'll talk about these later) while looking for some way to get an abundance of the brain's activity that swarms over the neurons, which in turn activates the neurons. The more this occurs, the better we feel, and the neurons are more likely to increase. This is how we change and grow.

When we learn and when we problem-solve, we feel better. It may come as a surprise to you to know that humor is a great way to stretch your brain. Humor can feed your brain in the same way that complex information does. In fact, the more you laugh or the funnier the information, the more neurons are activated.

Singer Reba McIntyre likes to repeat an old saying: "To succeed in life you need three things: a wishbone, a backbone, and a funny bone." Think back over the times in your life when you experienced a momentary discouraging setback. All seemed bleak as you counted up your losses. Bouncing back didn't seem like a viable option. Then, in the midst of the dark season, something struck you as funny. You heard a hilarious joke or watched a gut-splitting comedy, or just enjoyed a fun dinner out with really good friends where laughter was the main course of the evening. Suddenly, you felt better! For no apparent reason, your entire outlook changed, yet your circumstances were still the same. What just happened? Dr. Caroline Leaf explains:

> Many studies show why laughter deserves to be known as "the best medicine." It releases an instant flood of feel-good chemicals that boost the immune system and almost instantly reduce levels of stress hormones. For example, a really good belly laugh can make cortisol drop by 39% and adrenaline by 70%, while the "feel-good hormone," endorphin, increases by 29%. It can even make growth hormones skyrocket by 87%! Other research shows how laughter boosts your immune system by increasing immunity levels and disease-fighting cells...According to research,

laughing 100 to 200 times a day is equal to 10 minutes of rowing or jogging! Laugher quite literally dissolves distressing toxic emotions because you can't feel mad or sad when you laugh. Endorphins are released, making you feel so great and at peace that toxic thoughts can't get out of your brain fast enough.[2]

Wise King Solomon was right when he said, "A merry heart does good, like medicine, but a broken spirit dries the bones" (Proverbs 17:22 NKJV). Laughter is just another way the body is made to bounce.[3]

Your brain is amazing. It generates the equivalent of about ten to fifteen watts of energy—enough to power an LED bulb. Everything you've experienced thus far has altered the physical structure of your brain. Your family of origin, your culture, your friends, your work, every movie you've watched, every conversation you've had— these have all left their footprints in your nervous system. As you age, too, your brain's flexibility, and what you choose to expose it to, matters deeply.

Our brains don't need to remain as we've inherited them. We're now just discovering the tools to shape our own destiny. Who we become is up to us.[4]

So, the question is...How can you redesign your brain? We'll get to that—but first, let's take a tour of the body's most remarkable organ.

CHAPTER 2

Getting to Know Your Brain

What do you know about the most significant part of your body...your brain? Well, it controls you. How you think, how you feel, move, how you digest, how you disperse energy, and how you age.

I hope you'll like taking a tour. It's not a tour of another country nor a getaway—it's simply a look at the most important part of your body. We will uncover new ideas, new words, and new information. Many people today spend hours each week working their muscles and making sure they're in the best shape possible. Some stand in front of the mirror admiring their body and making sure every muscle is in top shape. My question is, Do you give your brain the same amount of care and attention? As one doctor said, "With your brain, you only get one in life, and medical science sees no prospects for transplants in the foreseeable future." It needs all the attention you can give to it. In order to do this, we need to understand our brain.

The Supervisor

The *frontal lobes* are one of the most important parts of your brain to understand. They're located directly behind the forehead and eyes, they're the largest set of lobes in your brain, and guess what…they're much larger than the frontal lobes of most animals. The frontal lobes receive information from all the other lobes. They gather the information and put it together to allow us to respond to the world in a meaningful way. Our frontal lobes have *executive functions*, meaning that they are where the supervision of many brain processes occur. If you want a supervisor, this is the place to find one. The good news is, the frontal lobes help us anticipate the results of situations, plan our actions, initiate responses, and use feedback from the world to stop or change our behaviors. You can actually renew and change these lobes by focusing on positive statements.

The bad news is, this is where the groundwork for anxiety and worry lies. These lobes anticipate and interpret situations, and anticipation often leads to anxiety. Because of our highly developed frontal lobes, humans have the ability to predict future events and imagine their consequences—unlike our pets, who seem to sleep peacefully without anticipating tomorrow's problems. Worry is an outgrowth of anticipation of negative outcomes in a situation.[1] We'll discuss this in greater detail in chapter 9.

The CEO

First of all, how many regions or lobes do you have in your brain? Four—that's all. They're easy to remember. The four words are *frontal*, *temporal*, *partial*, and *occipital*. The last two (partial and occipital) focus on your surroundings. The first half of your brain integrates what the body's senses take in and then analyzes that information before planning and carrying out decisions.

Every brain has a CEO, which directs what we do. We call this the frontal lobe and prefrontal cortex. This area of your brain has a number of important tasks to fulfill. What does it do? Consider this:

> The frontal lobes (the front half of the brain) are divided into three sections: the *motor* cortex, which controls the body's motor movements (such as jumping, chewing and wiggling your fingers); the *premotor* area, which is involved in planning those movements; and the *prefrontal cortex* (PFC), which directs executive functions like forethought, judgment, and impulse control. Short-term and working memories are first processed in the PFC as well.

> The prefrontal cortex enables us to learn from our mistakes and make plans. When the PFC is healthy, we behave consistently in ways that enable us to reach our goals. When it works as intended, we are organized, goal directed, thoughtful, empathetic and able to express feelings appropriately.

Do you know when yours is working?

> The PFC is often called the executive part of the brain and is closely associated with judgment, impulse control, attention span, self-monitoring, problem solving, and critical thinking. The prefrontal cortex is the brain's brake. It stops us from saying or doing stupid things.

Keep this in mind when you say something and regret it.

Not surprisingly, when the PFC isn't working as it should, problems such as impulsivity, distractibility, disorganization, faulty decision making, poor time management, and lack of empathy are evident.[2]

The Smoke Detector

The prefrontal cortex acts like the boss of all parts of the brain. It owns 30 percent of our brainscape, but it can be overruled by the other sections of our brain. That's where we get into trouble. The "smoke detector"—also known as the amygdala—can cause this trouble.

In the blink of the eye, the mere hint of a threat, rejection, or disappointment launches us into a high-speed preview chain of unstoppable catastrophes. Why is it that at the very moment when we need to think straight, our internal program makes us spin in spirals of worry?

Here's why: At the other end of the line when you perceive that initial reaction of distress is the *amygdala*, the brain's emotional response center. The amygdala is your round-the-clock surveillance system, overseeing your safety and in charge of the brain's 100 billion neurons and more.[3]

When you are making decisions, you may be affected by past choices, failure to look at consequences, and a "Why did I ever say that?" tendency. When pain hits, the logic of the CEO can be overruled by the Smoke Detector. One author describes what happens:

Who wants to listen to a CEO's logic when they're whirling in pain? It's like hitting our thumb with a hammer and being asked to recite the alphabet backwards. Our brains don't work that way. We need to start by calming our bodies first. Like frightened children, a panicked brain needs our mindful and focused attention to calm them down again. We can help them by literally pulling over to find a place to stop, catch our breath, and rest.

Calling a friend, taking several deep breaths, or sitting with our feet firmly planted on the ground are ways we can work toward calming our bodies down so we can think again. We can help our brains get back online by asking the CEO to name three objects in the room and identify their colors.[4]

The front part of your brain makes assessments. If the Smoke Detector alerts you, the CEO can restore your balance and let you know "it's a false alarm, so relax." Your stress level goes down. This section helps you to observe what is happening, predict what will happen if you take a certain action, and make a conscious choice.[5] As long as this portion of your brain is working as it should, you'll have the balance you want and you will be able to handle stress. But those who have post-traumatic stress disorder have a difficult time with this balance, and it's challenging to control emotions and impulses. When survival is at stake, we usually stop listening to the voices of reason. Your alarm portion has a purpose to protect you. But when the unexpected occurs, it overreacts. Your amygdala can actually prevent you from doing the very smart things that would be functional in a situation.[6]

You can also think of the amygdala like a dog. Now, you may be a person who enjoys dogs or perhaps not. Keep in mind the number of dog breeds is overwhelming. Some are bred to herd animals such as sheep or cattle. Others assist in the hunting process for sportsmen, by either flushing out the prey or pointing at the birds. Some are used for heavy labor such as huskies as they pull hundreds of pounds of sleds. Yet others use their heightened sense of smell for searching out drugs or cadavers or cancer. There are those used for protection; whereas, mine is more of a therapy dog.

The amygdala is like a dog, but unlike any just mentioned. It's a *watchdog* that's constantly on duty.

> The amygdala dictates where your attention goes, and at the least sign of danger it instantly mobilizes your body to fight or run for your life. Every ounce of energy you have becomes immediately available to defend your survival. That leaves very few ounces to do something rational like take a closer look at the situation to evaluate whether there really is a threat or just a temporary uncomfortable moment.[7]

Sometimes the amygdala lives its life as though it's on permanent sentry duty. And it's the site of emotional memory. It's the center-piece of our emotional system. It has a very refined memory system. It actually writes down memories of any trauma we experience. This system remembers sights, smells, and sounds of the worst experiences. It's not in the rational department. Don't expect that. This section of your brain doesn't operate on language or logic. It matches what it experienced and remembers with what occurs now. It couldn't care less whether its response makes sense or not. When you reexperience what you went through, it's because that watch-dog part of your brain went into action.[8]

At night you rest, but this portion continues to monitor your sensory information for any sign of threat. If there's an earthquake or a door slams shut or the cat knocks a vase to the floor, it will instantly detect the menacing noise. It then activates the connections to the startle response so that you leap out of bed—heart racing—ready to protect yourself.[9] It also becomes highly active during and while remembering a traumatic event. It controls your behavior. When you've been in trauma, it becomes hypersensitive and overreacts to normal stimuli.

But you can outsmart your overprotective brain by understanding that the amygdala is the default navigator. You can learn to avoid the urge to jump at every false alarm of doom and despair by taking back control and putting your voice of reason in the driver's seat.[10]

> If you can quickly recognize the amygdala's interruptions as unnecessary detours from the solid course you are on, you can reduce the time wasted on the negative. This allows you to stay focused on important things and get back on track with your life's path. It's an issue, but one that you can overcome.[11]

The Sentry

The Smoke Detector is concerned with your survival. And it is dependent upon another portion of the brain for feedback, as well as for preparing the body to handle the threat. I call this the Sentry.

The Sentry locates events in time and place and is connected to long-term memory storage. That's one of its biggest jobs. For example, when fear comes, it remembers where you were and what you were doing at the time. It is responsible for writing the story of the trauma, and it updates memory with new information. This is the portion of the brain that calms you down. It's also highly affected by trauma and can actually shrink in size.

This emotional system can't allow you to think about your reactions. That takes too much time. And it doesn't care if it makes you miserable. Under extreme stress, it shuts down the thinking part of your brain.[12] Has this ever happened to you?

The Smoke Detector triggers the mind and the body to prepare for action. When the danger is past, it returns to its normal state. These two little alarm glands are fairly good in picking up danger clues for you to access when you have experienced trauma.[13]

The Cook

We've given some practical names to some of the sections of the brain rather than the medical terminology to make it easier. We've already talked about the CEO (the prefrontal cortex) and the Smoke Detector (the amygdala). Now, let's turn our attention to the Cook.

It could be that over the years you've eaten homemade split pea soup (it's one of my favorites). It doesn't contain just peas, but numerous other ingredients: ham, peas, carrots, onions, celery, and broth. Could I eat all those ingredients individually and say I had split pea soup? No—the only way I can eat split pea soup is to stir all those ingredients together in a big pot. I need a cook to bring everything together!

A section of your brain called the thalamus acts like a cook. It takes all the perceptions which impact the brain and stirs them up into a blended autobiographical soup called "This is what's happening to me."

The Cook is a control tower for the senses. It receives incoming information through our senses of sight, smell, hearing, touch, and taste, and then passes it on to the other parts of the brain for processing. That's probably what it's doing right now. It's like a receiving department of a company, or a vacuum cleaner that sucks everything in, and it relays information to the portion where the memories are stored and activates those memories. If a negative memory is activated and alerted, then the emotional response that is carried back to the Cook (the relay stations) will be negative feelings.

Here is a picture of the brain and its various structures. This will show you how complex and unique your brain is. These are areas which are involved in the normal function of the brain.

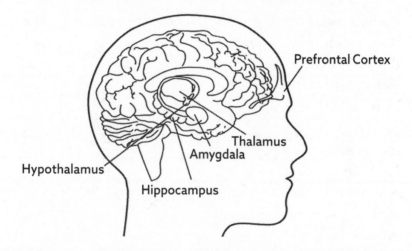

When everything is working as it should, we function as we should. But when one area is off, it can upset the others.

Sometimes, perhaps one of the best ways to think about the brain when it isn't working right is to think about it as an automatic transmission that isn't working properly. It's stuck in gear. I like the description in the book *Brain Lock*:

> You are cursed with a lousy manual transmission. In fact, even your manual doesn't work great. It's sticky. It's hard to shift, but, with effort, you *can* shift those gears yourself. It's not easy. It's hard work because the gearshift is stuck. But when they shift gears repeatedly, by consciously changing behaviors, they actually start to fix their transmission by changing the metabolism. They work around the glitch in the striatum. And the beauty of it is that this technique gets the transmission to slowly start working, automatically once again. It becomes easier to shift gears and to change behaviors as you keep working at it.[14]

It's not as difficult as it seems to understand the functioning as well as the structure of your brain. I've looked through several models. Having more than one to choose from allows you to select one you are comfortable with and relate to and understand. All are accurate in what they do and how they function. But the wording varies, and the more you work with the one you prefer, the deeper your level of understanding. At first, some things may seem complex, but the more you use the selection that appeals to you, the greater your understanding of enriching the health of your brain. You will become much more brain savvy, as it were.

I've tried to adapt what I have read and learned to make it easier for you to understand. It will be an adjustment because brain modeling is not a common choice of discussion. Most of us would fail a brain fluency test, but the more we understand about the brain, the more we'll be equipped to help it grow and change.

CHAPTER 3

Hardwired to Change

Let's go a different direction for a moment. Think about your brain. You have 100 billion nerve cells called neurons exploding with electrical charges 300 billion times per second. That's a lot!

Much of what is said in this book may be new to you. For example, have you ever heard of:

	Yes	No
The aging brain?		
Brain atrophy?		
Brain cell death?		
Brain freeze?		

All four of these can happen. What we need to do is to train our brains. We train them to create new, healthy brain cells. We need to repair our brain cells, maintaining our brains as they grow older. This is the process that fills the potholes on those streets so now the drive is smoother.

I'm sure you've heard the term *hardwired*. What it means is this: "a permanent feature in a computer by means of permanently connected circuits, so that it cannot be altered by software."[1] For decades we were told that our brains were hardwired like a computer—that the brain cells you had at birth were all that you would ever have—and that your brain was set up to function in what we call "predetermined ways." That was wrong. Your brain and mine is "soft-wired" and influenced by experience. The fact is, your brain is changing and repairing itself all the time. As John Arden puts it,

> In the last twenty years, there has been an overwhelming amount of evidence that the synapses are not hardwired but are changing all the time. This is what is meant by synaptic plasticity, or *neuroplasticity*. The synapses between the neurons are plastic. Neuroplasticity is what makes memory possible.
>
> Neuroplasticity illustrates the phrase, "Use it or lose it." When you use the synaptic connections that represent a skill, you strengthen them, and when you let the skill lie dormant, you weaken those connections. It's similar to the way that your muscles will weaken if you stop exercising.
>
> "Cells that fire together wire together" aptly describes the way your brain reorganizes when you have new experiences. The more you do something in a particular

way, use words with a specific accent, or remember something about your past, the more the neurons that fire together to make this happen will strengthen their connections. The more the neurons fire together, the more likely it is that they will fire together in the future.

When neurons fire together often, they begin to fire together at a quicker rate. This leads to increased efficiency, because there is more precision in the number of neurons that are required to do a particular skill.[2]

Were you aware that your brain carries on conversations with the various sections? It's true. I probably do this more than I realize. I've been accused of having a "hyper mind." It's usually creating something. Sometimes I'm aware of these conversations and sometimes not. We all have cells, but we're not always aware of the dialogues. These occur because of all the cells. One of those cells is called a neuron, and there is an abundance of them. How many? About 100 billion. And every neuron is connected to as many as 1,000 other neurons. And they are busy at work generating electric signals to stimulate other neurons. It's like an electrical switch has been turned on.

Neurons connect with one another, and these connections change as you learn. There are gaps between the neurons called synapses. It's difficult for me to think in visual terms when I hear *synapses*. But if you use the word *bridges*, that's something else. That I can see. It makes sense to me. *Bridges.*

Messages go across these bridges to get other neurons to fire. They activate them. There are about 60 types of neurotransmitters in the brain—some get you excited, and some bring you down.

A key word to remember is *neuroplasticity*. How important is this? It's critical. This makes memory possible. It really means that the bridges between the neurons are plastic. When you change your synapses, you remember something new. When you remember something new, you are reviving your brain. *The more you do something new, the more your brain changes.*

Have you had the experience of driving on a bridge and feeling the bridge lift gently up and down? If it didn't have that flexibility, the bridge would break. These bridges in your brain are the same. They are able to move and change so we can learn new things.

When I try playing a new song on the piano, my brain changes. My brain is not stuck in a certain way. It can grow. Just think! At the end of a day, you can look at yourself in the mirror and say, "My brain grew today! It's different." The more you do something in a certain way, the more neurons fire together, and the more likely you will do it in the same way. If I play one song several times on the piano, when I sit down to play it again, it's more likely that it will come back to me more easily and quickly. My brain also changes and grows when I imagine playing the song. As one writer puts it,

> Not only does behavior change the structure of the brain through neuroplasticity, just thinking about or imagining particular behaviors can change brain structure as well. For example, researchers have shown that simply imagining a session of piano practice contributes to neuroplasticity in the area of the brain associated with the finger movements of playing the piano. Thus, mental practice alone contributes to the rewiring of the brain.[3]

Your brain was designed by a God of love, joy, and peace. Have you ever wondered, when you have a joyful thought, why you suddenly begin to feel joyful all over? Your brain is secreting a joy chemical down your brain stem into your heart, and it's circulating through the arteries of your body. Have you ever been separated from a loved one for an extended period of time, and at the moment of reunion you are overwhelmed with the emotion of love? A love chemical has been secreted down your brain stem into your heart and then pumped through your body. Your entire nervous system is overwhelmed with love.

Have you ever felt stressed and pressured, stopped to pray, and suddenly felt peace in the midst of the storm? A peace chemical is fulfilling its God-given purpose recorded in Scripture: "You will keep him in perfect peace, whose mind is stayed on You, because he trusts in You" (Isaiah 26:3 NKJV). Did you catch that? The mind that is at peace is focused on God.

> Why, then, do you react physically when you are living in fear of the future? Why do you weave that proverbial knot in your stomach, find sleep difficult, and generally become irritable when you are experiencing the stress of fear? When you suffer loss and struggle with the fear of failure and doubt, how can you press on regardless of your circumstances?[4]

> You are not a victim of biology. God has given us a design of hope; we can switch on our brains, renew our minds, change and heal…The implications of this are obvious; we need to take responsibility for our choices and subsequent words, actions and behaviors. We can't blame anyone else.[5]

Challenge Your Mind

My brother completed a crossword puzzle daily for 60 years. I've learned not to play Scrabble with him since his vocabulary is so extensive. As I've said before, I continue to play the piano several times a week but search for new pieces and take "lessons" by listening to performers on CD and then using what I've learned to improve. Sometimes the muscles in my hands don't respond to what my brain is telling them, but in time and with practice, they do get better.

More and more studies are showing how we can learn in our seventies and eighties. Auditory memory programs and other brain-exercise programs slow down age-related cognitive decline and lead to better overall functioning. Some people have been able to turn their memory clock back ten to twenty years. There are even exercises to affect specific sections of the brain.

We're deeply affected by our beliefs and attitudes. We could look at this and say, "I don't believe it" or "It won't work for me." How will you know unless you give it a real try?

Remember: We have a choice as to how we age. As one writer puts it, "There are things you *can* do to tip the odds of memory preservation versus decline decidedly in your favor. You are *not* destined to become forgetful."[6] Let me repeat this: You are *not* destined to be forgetful.

As you mature through the teen years and into your twenties, 50 percent of your synapses will be pared back. By now you know what a synapse is—remember the bridge.

Which synapses stay and which go? When a synapse successfully participates in a circuit, it is strengthened. Synapses that aren't used are weakened and eventually eliminated, just as with paths in a forest. You lose the connections that you don't use.

Listening to or playing music can activate the motor cortex (touching a piano key or guitar string), the auditory cortex (hearing the notes you make), and the emotional center, or limbic system (feeling moved by a beautiful passage).

Rebuilding Your Brain

I've had people tell me, "Norm, I'd like to get the most out of my brain. I want it to work for me...not against me. I've read articles about the brain and know that it's possible." It's true—you can rewire your brain, so you get the most out of your life and your daily experience.

The "consolidation of adulthood" takes place between the ages of 20 and 40, This is when the downpour of hormones subsides and brain chemical levels begin to stabilize. The brain reorganizes itself to function more effectively. This is when we are at our peak mental performance. Most adults tend to establish their careers, start families, and generally settle down at this point. But then some changes begin to occur. We call this hormonal change.

What happens to us during this time? It's like we pull ourselves together during the ages of 20 to 40. It's like we've peaked, and then there is a slow but steady functional decline. Attention wanders, thinking slows, and anxiety increases. And then each decade thereafter, mild cognitive impairment (MCI) begins as brain speed and voltage are lost. By the time you and I are 70, many of us have reached what is called low-voltage dementia. Brain cells are no longer repairing themselves, memory retention is destroyed, and processing speed undergoes a very slow death.

All cognitive functions—your creativity, intelligence, and ability to remember, communicate, concentrate, or recall—are affected by the anatomy and chemistry of the brain, first by your brain's processing speed, and then by the presence and flow of its electrical energy. I know that's a mouthful. Here's the problem. These functions naturally decline with age as brain cells die off, neuronal connections become short-circuited, and cerebrospinal fluid decreases.

Unfortunately, you will notice that your body begins to age

before you realize that your brain speed has changed. (It's not the mirror that has changed—you have.)

The gradual, progressive cognitive decline associated with an aging brain exists on a continuum, just like the one that links minor allergies to severe asthma. When cognitive impairment is sufficiently great, such that there is interference with daily functions, you may be diagnosed with the third and final stage: dementia. This is not something you look forward to!

Pre-MCI stages can begin a full 20 years before significant symptoms occur. We now know that by the age of 40, 25 to 50 percent of Americans are already affected by MCI, even though less than one percent will show any symptoms. Again, this is why it is so critical to maintain that younger 30-year-old brain for the rest of your life.

The Warning Signs of MCI

Most people who are suffering from MCI can still function in daily activities but may be less efficient or accurate. Three warning signs of MCI are:

- Losing things often
- Forgetting to go to events or appointments
- Having more trouble coming up with words than other people your same age

Let's talk now about memory loss. When it comes to our memory, many people wonder, "Am I losing it?" When you realize that your memory isn't as sharp as it once was, you might think, "There goes the brain." But it's part of our future. Do you know what is the first thing to go in our memory? If you guessed "someone's name," you're right. The phrase "I'll never forget old what's-his-name" is a common expression.

We only have a limited storage department for memory, and names are the first to go. We are more prone to remember events, but as we age, we remember events of long ago differently. Memories of childhood trauma may be distorted.

As you age, so does your brain. You can expect to experience changes in your memory and attention as you age. You and I will actually experience a loss of brainpower. The older we get, the less capable we are. We're concerned about losing our minds.

Your brain actually atrophies in the same way your muscles do when you fail to exercise. Have you ever heard of the shrinking brain? Without proper care, blood flow to the brain can decrease.

But some of us experience a cognitive reserve. We stay sharp mentally. Why? Here's how one report puts it:

> Research has supported the concept that individuals can create a "buffer" of sorts that protects them from the cognitive deficits seen with age- or disease-related brain changes. This buffer is thought to be as result of a greater proliferation of and connection between neurons in the brain in response to cognitively stimulating experiences.
>
> Factors like education, an intellectually challenging career, exercise, and mentally and socially stimulating activities are thought to contribute to cognitive reserve. Research suggests people with more cognitive reserve are better able to stave off the degenerative brain changes associated with dementia, or to maintain cognition in the face of those changes.[7]

As I age, I wonder about my mental ability. Most of the time I remember, but like most of those my age, I have concerns. But our bodies are designed for self-repair—including our brains! MCI is like a wound inside the brain, and we can teach it to repair itself just like a cut on a finger. Our brain doesn't have to deteriorate if we take care of it and treat it well. There is so much we can do to keep our brain functional.

As Gail Sheehy wrote,

> Because most seniors accept outdated cultural poll studies about "dotty old people," they underestimate their mental skills, which are particularly high in reasoning and verbal expression, and try to evade intellectual tasks—exactly the opposite of what they should do to stay sharp. Their pessimism often leads to a premature and unnecessary dependence on others—spouses or children or their doctors.
>
> People who develop the discipline of daily mental exercise—reading newspapers instead of only passively ingesting TV news, noodling over the crossword puzzle every day, keeping journals, balancing their checkbook, and reading the fine print on insurance forms, etc.—are preparing themselves...
>
> [They] can become distinguished today by belonging to the new aristocracy of successful aging...[Their] added years offer an opportunity to display a great generosity of mind and soul, to forgive former enemies or to show dignity of conception in composing a thought, a poem, an expression of any sort that helps illuminate the path for others coming behind them...
>
> Your immune system needs to be signaled that you believe your life is worth fighting for. Again, even if you

don't know what will give your life meaning at this stage, the very process of searching and working at it, every day, is a healing process, because it is opening up hope.[8]

There are numerous options to reverse the deterioration of our brain. This brief look is just an introduction to help you expand your knowledge and begin the process of moving forward to have a healthy brain. I will be suggesting numerous steps, but hopefully won't overload you. It's important to remember the steps and implement them.

The first step is early detection. You may need some help in evaluating where you are at this time.

The second step is making lasting lifestyle changes and clearing out the clutter of your mind.

Before we dive into those steps, though, remember: If you enrich your brain, you'll enrich your whole life.

DID YOU KNOW?

- There are no pain receptors in the brain, so the brain can feel no pain.
- The brain contains 100,000 miles of blood vessels.
- The cerebral cortex grows thicker as you learn to use it.
- Reading aloud and talking often to a young child promotes brain development.
- Children who learn two languages before the age of five have a much denser gray matter as adults.
- The brain can live for four to six minutes without oxygen, and then it begins to die. No oxygen for five to ten minutes will result in permanent brain damage.

- Excessive stress has shown to change brain cells, brain structure, and brain function.
- Five minutes after a dream, half of the dream is forgotten. Ten minutes after a dream, over 90 percent is forgotten. Write down your dreams immediately if you want to remember them.
- Juggling has shown to change the brain in as little as seven days.
- Laughing at a joke is no simple task! It requires activity in five different areas of the brain.
- Music lessons have been shown to considerably boost brain organization and ability in both children and adults.
- The average number of thoughts that humans are believed to experience each day is 70,000.
- Those who are left-handed or ambidextrous have a corpus callosum (the part of the brain that bridges the two halves) that is about 11 percent larger than those who are right-handed.
- Famous for knowing all the London streets by heart, London taxi drivers have a larger than normal hippocampus, especially the drivers who have been on the job longest. The study suggests that as people memorize more and more information, this part of their brain continues to grow.[9]
- By the age of seven, our first memories are almost entirely erased. A teen recalls no more of her early childhood than a 50-year-old.[10]

CHAPTER 4

The Basics of Brain Refreshment

I need to admit something: I'm biased. It probably shows. I emphasize certain steps above others for enriching your brain, but it doesn't mean that what I choose to emphasize is more important and more significant than what I left out.

It's important to like, enjoy, be challenged by, or be amazed by whatever we choose to focus upon. How do we overcome our bent or our bias? Focus on what you are interested in or are drawn to, if possible, and spend 70 percent of your time there and 30 percent of your time elsewhere. Will it work? For some people it will, for others not. But it's worth a try.

Diet

What about what we eat? Our brains are very much impacted by what we eat—good or bad. Books and books and books have been written about what we ingest. The bottom line is this: The Western diet, as it is called, is not healthy. Look at what you eat. All I ask is for you to keep track of whatever you eat and drink for one month. The results may speak for themselves. It's not always what you eat but what is in what you eat.

If you have never read about the Mediterranean diet, you're in for a treat. Perhaps not in the way you think of treats, but this diet could open an entirely new dimension of taste and substance. Unlike our Western diets, meals for the Mediterranean diet are built around plant-based foods with moderate amounts of dairy, poultry, and seafood. Research has shown that healthful eating such as found with the Mediterranean diet improves cognition, memory, and brain volume and offers a protective effect on brain health.[1]

Think fruit with me. Which fruits are the best for you? Blueberries are at the top of the list. Strawberries are also credited with preventative capabilities, even reducing the onset of cancer. And my favorite—raspberries—are thought to protect the brain from oxidative stress and help reduce the effects of age-related conditions such as dementia. Yes, these berries may cost a bit more, but compare the food value of these with all of the empty food products we ingest.

But the most important part of your diet is available to you at a minimal cost. Water! Most of us don't drink enough. Your body is 60 percent water, but your brain is 75 percent! The electrolytes are suspended in our body's fluid, and we need water to keep the system functioning.

When we are well hydrated, our brains are cushioned the way

they're supposed to be, and our central nervous system can function well as it sends electrical signals along nerve pathways. With plenty of water in our system, our brains can concentrate. We are more alert and cheerful. Our memory is sharper, and we are less likely to experience anxiety and depressive thoughts.

Use your weight as a guide. Spread out your liquid intake throughout the day.

Not only does drinking water help enhance the brain, wading or swimming does also. How? Wading or swimming improves cerebrovascular health, the flow of useful fluids throughout circulatory systems. It increases the blood flow to the brain, as well as decreasing depression. As brain chemicals are stimulated, your mood is elevated. There are many exercise programs that you can discover to meet your needs.

Mental Gymnastics

By now, you're probably wondering, "When are we going to get to the brain games?" Mental gymnastics stimulate the brain, and the growth of brain cells is encouraged. Brain games are all around us, including apps on our phones. Go to the Internet or bookstores, and you will be overwhelmed by the number of games you will find.

You and I are creatures of habit. We're comfortable with the routine in our life. And there is nothing wrong with that. And I'm not suggesting that you change your habits and routines. But why not add something new for your brain's sake? Studies show that when you learn something new, your memory is improved not just immediately but even a year later. What have you learned that is new and mentally challenging in the last year? It's not that you have to drop the familiar and routine, but add on to it. Consider these questions:

What have I learned that's new in the last year?

_____

_____

_____

What are the obstacles to maintaining this?

_____

_____

_____

This is what I will do to overcome obstacles:

_____

_____

_____

Another way to enhance your brain is by refreshing it—your brain *can* be refreshed. It will take time, commitment, and discipline. Mental exercise is as important as diet and physical exercise for keeping your body and brain strong. You may have already discovered something that works. That's great. Be open to something new.

Here is a list of activities that have been shown to make a difference. I've had a number of people read the suggestions and say, "But I've been doing many of these for much of my life." If so, be thankful since you've been taking good care of your brain without knowing it. Which of these suggestions are already a part of your life, and which ones can you incorporate into your daily routines?

Music

Music has tremendous power. Your mind, feelings, and behavior are impacted by the music you hear, especially as you watch a movie or a TV show. It can stir us up or have a calming effect. Listening can actually make long-term changes to your brain, and it may stimulate neurogenesis. Listening, playing, singing, and even dancing promote brain health. Why? Often the music intensifies our memories, stimulating and synchronizing the left and right hemispheres. Those who listen to their favorite music repeatedly even report better moods.

Use music to enhance your mind. There has been significant research suggesting that both learning to play music and listening to music, especially classical music, can enhance memory and mood. Classical musical also enhances memory and cognitive function.[2] For example, listening to Mozart or Strauss for just 25 minutes a day has been shown to lower blood pressure and the stress hormone cortisol.[3] Listening to peaceful and joyful music lowered anxiety and depression.[4] Learning to play music helped to increase the size of the hippocampus.[5] Sit down at your piano! Stevie Wonder once said, "Music, at its essence, is what gives us memories." Research shows that listening to happy or peaceful music leads to the recall of positive memories, while listening to frightening or sad music dredges up most negative memories.[6] Music matters.

I can't say enough about the value of music, especially the piano. Research studies abound. After a year or two of practicing, motor and auditory skill are increased, and actual structural changes in the brain can be observed. Practice, practice, and then practice some more.

Memory journaling

You're probably aware that your emotions and moods can affect what you remember. You remember less if your memory is a negative one, and more if the memory is pleasant. You will recall pleasant information more accurately and quicker. Your brain is wired to retain pleasant memories longer and unpleasant ones fade faster.[7]

Have you heard of a memory journal? It helps to activate the creative side of your brain. Some share what they write on a blog or on social media. If you'd like to make your memories public, one writer notes,

> Be sure you feel comfortable with others reading what you post. If not, consider just posting those parts of your journal anyone can read and keep the other parts offline. A good way to make the distinction is to keep personal observations and thoughts about yourself in your private offline journal; but if you have any insights about what you can do to improve your memory—which could be useful for anyone else—by all means, post them for all to see.[8]

Prior to creating your journal, here are some questions to guide you:

1. My overall goal (what you hope to achieve by the end of 30 days)

2. My goals for today (the areas of memory improvement you are focusing on now)

3. My memory successes (specific incidents, experiences, and observations where you enjoyed a notable, outstanding, or unexpected success)

4. My memory lapses (specific times when you found you weren't able to recall or recognize something at all or where you remembered it incorrectly)

5. Trends and patterns (types of things you are likely to remember, types of things you find you often forget or remember incorrectly)

6. Memory improvements (things you find you can remember now that you didn't before)

7. Memory challenges (things that you are continuing to find especially difficult to remember)

8. Memory insights (ideas and tips you have gained from your own experiences in trying to remember things or in keeping this journal, plus ideas and tips you have gained from your reading or from others—including talking to people or from radio or TV)[9]

Memorization

Your brain needs you to memorize. We have short-term memory and long-term. Whatever you choose to memorize, your brain thanks you. When you're working on memorizing, try repeating the selection out loud again and again.

New people and places

Dedicate yourself to new learning. Devote just 15 minutes a day to a new hobby, activity, or subject matter. As in school or business, commitment is critical if you want to reap the benefits.

Community-dwelling seniors who took just a few weeks of cognitive training experienced significantly improved reasoning and speed of processing skills, as well as fewer difficulties with the activities of daily living ten years later, compared with those who didn't get such training.[10]

Take a class and learn something new. Community colleges and online groups offer low-cost courses. Challenge your brain to learn novel and interesting things by taking a class that is unrelated to your work or daily life. Working with modeling clay or Play-Doh can help children or adults develop new neural connections, as well as agility and hand-brain coordination.

Cross-train at work. Learning someone else's job or even switching jobs for several weeks provides workers with better skills and brain function and may offer the employer greater flexibility.

Limit television. Adults who watch more than two hours of TV a day have a significantly higher risk of Alzheimer's disease. Watching TV is usually a "no brain activity" unless it is an educational program.

Alter daily routines to stimulate new parts of your brain. Do the opposite of what feels natural to activate the other side of your brain and gain access to both hemispheres. When you write, dress, brush your teeth, set the table, shoot baskets, play ping pong, or use your computer mouse, use your nondominant hand. These changes make your brain feel uncomfortable—in essence, breaking the patterned routine in your life and challenging your brain to make new connections.

Travel to new and interesting places. Exposing the brain to unique experiences, scents, sights, and people strengthens your brain. What would be new for you?

Develop friendships with smart people. You become like the people you hang out with. You can trade ideas, get new perspectives, and generally stretch your mind if you are surrounded by fascinating folks. Most of us know that to improve when playing any game, we have to play with people who are better than we are. The same principle holds true in pushing your brain to new heights. Spend time with people who challenge you.

Finally, treat learning problems. Numerous studies show that better-educated people are at a lower risk of developing Alzheimer's disease and cognitive decline. Yet, millions of people struggle with learning, despite having normal or even high intelligence. Often these difficulties stem from ADD or other learning issues. Recognizing and addressing these problems are essential to making "lifelong learning" a reality. You can take an online test to help you determine whether you have ADD at www.amenclinics.com.[11]

See like a camera, listen like a recorder

This exercise will help you to observe or listen more accurately and completely in everyday situations. This technique can be used wherever you are—it's especially ideal for parties, business networking meetings, and other important occasions where you want to be sure to remember things accurately. Also, you can use this technique to practice and sharpen your skills when you're waiting in line, traveling in a bus, in a theater lobby at intermission, and in places where you are waiting for something to happen.

Simply imagine you are a camera and take a picture of what you see. Or imagine you are a recorder taping a conversation. Or focus on both sight and sound and imagine videotaping what you see and hear.

After you have finished, stop and look away or close your eyes for a few seconds, and focus on what you have seen or heard. If you have taken a picture, visualize it intently in your mind's eye and concentrate. Focus on the details in the picture. Who do you see? What do you see? What colors do you notice? What objects are in the room? What are the people wearing?

Then, open your eyes or look back at the scene and compare your mental picture with what you see now. What was missing? Did you add anything that wasn't there? What did you observe incorrectly? The more you do this, the more accurate your picture will be.

If you tried listening like a recorder, replay what you have heard in your mind. What were people talking about? What surrounding noises did you hear? You won't be able to hear these conversations or sounds again, but you can get a sense of how much detail you were able to pick up. The more you practice, the more fully you will hear.

If you have imagined yourself as a film camera, review both the pictures and sounds.[12]

Breathe deep

One of the ways of calming your mind is through deep breathing exercises. I have participated in a number of them, and they are quite effective. One of the most helpful books is *Power Over Panic* by Bronwyn Fox. The following is from this resource. The author discusses an exercise described as diaphragmatic breathing.

> Football players have a saying they use often, "A good defense makes a good offense." In our game plan to win against worry and anxiety, diaphragmatic or deep breathing is the first line of defense.

> Deep breathing doesn't cost anything, but it does take a little time and effort to practice. It should be utilized twice a day for ten minutes each time and as needed throughout the day to condition the body to relax. Sometimes a person may need to do these exercises for a period of a month or longer before relief begins. Consistency in practicing is critical to helping your body relax.

> No matter how consistent you are, however, deep breathing will not be effective unless you breathe from your diaphragm. Most people over five years old tend to be self-conscious about letting their abdomen relax

and "hang out" and have lost the ability to breathe in this healthy way. If your tummy is not going out on your inhale and in on exhale, you're not breathing correctly. To practice this technique, lie on the floor and put a book on your abdomen directly under your ribcage. When you inhale, the book should rise and when you exhale it will come down again.

Deep breathing needs to be incorporated into your lifestyle as a daily habit. It should also be used when you become nervous and overwhelmed during the course of the day. If you become anxious before speaking, deep breathing is a natural process that can be done on the way to the podium. If anxiety develops when you're driving, pull to the side of the road and begin the process. If your husband is upset with you, you can ask for a time out and follow this simple process before returning to the conversation. Deep breathing is a simple way to manage anxiety and worry and retrain your body to relax.[13]

Are there any kinds of experiences which impact our brain more than others? What really resonates in your brain most will be the emotional events that are personally meaningful. They are usually accompanied with higher levels of arousal and actuate a physical reaction. So, as these events occur, they create neuroplastic changes and lock in the memory. A basic principle is this: If you want to remember something, become emotionally involved in it.[14] Whether it's joining a new community class or traveling somewhere new, give it your all!

CHAPTER 5

Right and Left

Let's consider some details about your brain.

We all know (or should) about the differences in the male-female brain. Overall, men tend to have larger brains, but women have a greater density in the language areas, as well as the decision-making portions of the brain and the memory portion. Their emotional circuitry reaction is often larger as well. Perhaps your response is, "I knew that" or "Aha! I knew there was some reason for that!"

The left and the right sides of the brain are connected, communicating through a series of nerve bundles. These connections bring together the emotional and thinking sides of our existence. Women have up to 20 to 40 percent more of these nerve bundles than men, which means that they are better able to use both sides of their brain at the same time. Men, meanwhile, have to switch from one side of the brain to the other, depending upon what they need.

Someone described the differences in this way: A woman's brain is like a massive freeway system with roads going every which way; a man's brain is more like a one-way dirt road! Women can enjoy more cross talk between both sides of the brain, since they use their brains holistically. This is why they can handle several tasks at one time and can read earlier than boys. However, we need the function of both sides to have balance and to derive the most out of life. Bill and Pam Farrel describe it this way:

> Men are like waffles—men process life in boxes. If you look at the top of a waffle, you see a collection of boxes separated by walls. The boxes are all separate from each other and make convenient holding places. That is typically how men process life. His thinking is divided up into boxes that have room for one issue and one issue only. The first issue of life goes in the first box, the second goes in the second box, and so on. The typical man lives in one box at a time and one box only. As a result, when a man is at work, he is at work. When he is in the garage tinkering around, he is in the garage tinkering. When he is watching TV, he is simply watching TV. That is why he looks as though he is in a trance and can ignore everything else going on around him. Social scientists call this "compartmentalizing"—that is, separating life and responsibilities into different compartments.

> As men mature, they improve in their ability to jump from one box to another. They can move from compartment to compartment faster than they used to,

which creates a pretty good imitation of multitasking. In reality, they're just jumping out of boxes at a quicker pace.

A man will strategically organize his life in boxes and then spend most of his time in the boxes *he can succeed in.* This is such a strong motivation for him, that he will seek out the boxes that work and ignore the boxes that confuse him or make him feel like a failure. For instance, a man whose career holds the possibility of success will spend more and more time at work at the expense of other priorities.

Women process information more like a plate of pasta. If you look at a serving of spaghetti, you'll notice there are lots of individual noodles, and you might even switch in another noodle seamlessly. That is how women handle life. Every thought and issue is connected to every other thought and issue in some way. Life is much more connected, much more of a process for women than men.[1]

Emotions and the Brain

You are an emotional creation. Be thankful for this. God created you and how you function. And the most amazing and perhaps least understood part of us is our brain. You may think, "I'm not influenced by my emotions that much. I'm a thinking, rational being." That may be true. But your brain and mine are created in such a way that no information gets through to the rational, thinking part of your brain without passing through the area of your brain where your emotions originate. And believe it or not, your emotions color that information and also determine how much attention is paid to it.

Have you ever been hijacked? Your answer is probably, "No, of course not." A more accurate answer is probably, "Yes, I have." Many of us have, but we didn't realize it. Whenever we experience the unexpected, that possibility is there. The alarm section is responsible for this.

There is a portion of your brain that's always on the alert for the worst! It's like a radar constantly searching. If there is the slightest indication of a problem or pain or the unthinkable, it turns on its switch and wants to get into action. Sometimes this portion of your brain is referred to as the alarm section or smoke detector. Its real name is the amygdala, but who wants to try to remember that!

When your emotional side (the right) is highly activated, you tend to shut down the thinking or rational (the left) side. It's like you're caught in an emotional grip or vise and you insist that your thinking, even though highly influenced by your emotions, is accurate and logical; whereas, in reality, it may not be. Someone described it as if your emotions hijacked your thinking or the rational side of your brain.

Based on your life's experiences, you may develop an emotional allergy, which is an intense reactivity to a situation that is similar to an event that was painful in your past but is *not* the same situation in the present.

This intense reaction functions as if we are emotionally allergic. If there is one hint in the present of what happened in the past, we believe the same painful outcome will occur even when our present situation is quite different.

This is important to remember. For you to move forward, you will need to turn off one section of your brain (the alarm and its painful memories) and turn on the neo-cortex frontal lobes. Do you know how to do this? You will; it's possible, and this can change your life.

Our brains create explanations and then continue to look for them in other situations as a way of keeping us safe. You will hear this in phrases again and again. We look for *safety*. Consider these experiences that plague many:

Abandonment: "I'll end up alone."

Deprivation: "My needs won't be met."

Subjugation: "It's always your way, not mine."

Mistrust: "They're out to get me."

Unlovability: "I'm not lovable."

Exclusion: "I'm always left out."

Vulnerability: "I'm responsible but can't control the situation, so I feel overwhelmed and worry excessively."

Failure: "I'm not good enough."

Entitlement: "I'm special, so rules don't apply to me."

Perfection: "I have to do everything perfectly."

It's as though these are tattooed on our brain.

Who can live up to these? I can't.

Do you relate to any of these? If so, do you remember their origin?

Has anyone ever said, "Quit responding with your emotions. Just think about this, and you'll respond better as well as calm down"? Does this work? No, it doesn't, and it won't.

Have you heard of *brain shifting*? Probably not. It occurs all the time, sometimes purposely and sometimes not. Brain scans have been used to help understand our functioning. Scans show that images of past trauma, such as flashbacks, activate the right side of our brain (the emotional or feelings side) and thoughts the left or thinking side. Each side of the brain speaks a different language.

Under ordinary circumstances, the two sides of the brain work together more or less smoothly, even in people who might be said to favor one side over the other. However, having one side or the other shut down, even temporarily, or having one side cut off entirely (as sometimes happens in brain surgery) is disabling.

When something reminds a traumatized person of the past, their right brain reacts as if the traumatic event were happening right now, in the present. But because their left brain is not working very well, they may not be aware that they're reexperiencing and reenacting the past—they're furious, terrified, enraged, ashamed, or frozen. "What is going on?" is their cry. After the emotional storm passes, they may even look for something or somebody to blame for it. They think they behaved the way they did because of what someone else did. When they cool down, they hopefully can admit their mistake. However, trauma interferes with this kind of awareness.[2] Keep that in mind when the above happens. There's nothing wrong with you. It's the result of the unexpected.

Our brain generates emotions. We need these. And we were created as emotional beings. You're not limited emotionally, but you benefit from your emotions. But keep this in mind: When you are emotionally free rather than imprisoned, you will have more resources to handle the difficult situations that occur. Perhaps you're bound up emotionally because of what you experienced as a child, such as being told, "Don't cry," or "Stuff your feelings." You may have been damaged or hurt as a child emotionally, and this hinders you. We have a choice—we can live in the past as a victim, or we can assume a new level of responsibility and take charge. People who do this are referred to as overcomers. Those who don't are, in some ways, prisoners in their own jail. Emotions are part of our life.

We need them—but in balance. Someone said emotion and reason work like a seesaw. The stronger your emotions, the more difficult it is to think clearly. But this is where the seesaw comes in. It can work the other way as well. If you're thinking straight, sometimes this process can override your emotions.

> Your brain is amazing. Do you know the brain can indeed be rewired? It can expand the area that is wired to move the fingers, forging new connections that underpin the dexterity of an accomplished violinist. It can activate long-dormant wires and run new cables like an electrician bringing an old house up to code, so that regions that once saw can instead feel or hear. It can quiet circuits that once crackled with the aberrant activity that characterizes depression and cut pathological connections that keep the brain in the *oh-no-something-is-wrong* state that marks obsessive-compulsive disorder. The adult brain, in short, retains much of the plasticity of the developing brain, including the power to repair damaged regions, to grow new neurons, to rezone regions that performed one task and have them assume a new task, to change the circuitry that weaves neurons into the networks that allow us to remember, feel, suffer, think, imagine, and dream.[3]

CHAPTER 6

Who You Are Inside

Let's get practical. I've spent over 50 years helping people, in one way or another, discover who they are and why they are the way they are. I've heard questions like, "Why do I do what I do?" or "Why am I so different from...?" or "Is it possible for me to change and respond like other people do?" Well, you've probably guessed it. Much of who we are has to do with our brain.

We're going to look at the uniqueness of our personality—or why you are the way you are! Who are you, and why are you that way? Consider these characteristics:

Have you ever been frustrated with another person because they always seem preoccupied with heaven-only-knows-what? It's your brain and their brain.

Do you start the day with great intentions to get a few specific things done but get distracted? Again, it's your brain.

Have you ever been excited about going to a group so that you can spend time with a lot of your friends, but the friend you're going with complains about having to endure another evening of shallow conversation? You each have your brain to thank!

Does it ever surprise you that people view you as insensitive and uncaring, when deep down inside you are very sensitive and care deeply for others? You just don't show it.

Nowhere is the breadth of God's creativity more evident than in humankind. No two of us are exactly alike. Even identical twins can have opposite personalities. Each of us has a combination of gifts, talents, attitudes, beliefs, needs, and wants that is different from anyone else's. That's part of what makes life so exciting. It's all right to be different!

Your Relationship with You

What type of relationship do you have with yourself? The answer may be the key to who we are and where we're going over the next few years. The relationship we have with ourselves can lead to satisfaction, security, and contentment, as well as an increasing depth of our relationship with Jesus. But our relationship with self can also lead to feelings of isolation, loneliness, and disconnection.

I remember Janice. She shared openly about her relationship with herself. When anyone met her, they were usually impressed with how secure and confident she appeared. It was evident in her work and her relationship with others, but in time as she became more transparent, she dropped her façade and opened her life. She said, "What you see is not who I really am. I engage in cover-up, so others won't know the real me. Actually, the best way for me to describe who I am inside is I feel fragmented." When I heard this, the picture that came to mind was a huge boulder with cracks running through it. This feeling of fragmentation can lead to emotional and physical isolation. It's not uncommon, then, to feel that others misunderstand you.

Do others really know you? Perhaps the question is, Do you really know you? Many feel alone and isolated from others—and worse, feeling disconnected in some way from themselves.

Jim gave me a description that many seem to relate to. He said, "Some days I feel disconnected inside of myself. In fact, it doesn't feel like my brain is fully connected." Is that possible? To have your brain in pieces or fragments?

I've heard some people say they feel as though their brain is in pieces. Perhaps this description may apply to you in some way.

> As you know your brain is made up of two major parts. You have the logical left side of your brain that may successfully maintain in focus on the tasks of daily living, allowing you to stay in your job and make it through your day-to-day routine. However, the more experiential right side of your brain, where the majority of your memories are stored, may remain in a continued state of fear, vulnerability, or shame. You may attempt to ignore this part. You may attempt to ignore this part of you in favor of just getting through your day, which is certainly understandable but unfortunately leads to further fragmentation and self-alienation. You may also judge these emotional responses in yourself as negative or weak, thus attempting to further distance yourself from your experiences and labeling them as "not the real me." Unfortunately,

drowning parts of yourself will only lead to feeling more unsafe and unsettled within your own skin.[1]

Here are some questions, which may help you look at yourself.

What is your fear of what's inside of you?

_____

_____

_____

How do you engage your brain at this time?

_____

_____

_____

Who do you want to be?

_____

_____

_____

How do you want to be?

_____

_____

_____

How do you get along with yourself?

_____

_____

_____

The Building Blocks of Personality

If you have ever observed families with more than one child, you've probably been amazed that children from the same gene pool, raised by the same parents, in the same neighborhood, eating the same diet, going to the same school and church, can be totally different. What accounts for these differences? A major reason is the brain.

Why do some people love to be alone for hours on end, and others go crazy if people aren't around? Why does one person always come up with new ideas and invent things, while another is content to use things the way they're "supposed" to be used? Why do some people like to talk things out, while others prefer to work it out for themselves and then talk about it? Why does one person welcome a new person in a group, and another want to keep membership exclusive? How can some people read a book for an hour without being bored or distracted, while others start climbing the wall after only ten minutes? Why do some people take pride in having a clean and neat office, while other offices appear as if they've been used for nuclear testing?

In Psalm 139:14, we read, "Thank you for making me so wonderfully complex! It is amazing to think about. Your workmanship is marvelous—and how well I know it" (TLB). The Bible clearly teaches that every person is made in the image of God and is of infinite worth and value. Differences in personality types or temperament are the reason you see such variations in people.

Personality type consists of several inborn preferences or tendencies that have a strong impact on how we develop as individuals. Each of us begins life with a small number of inherited personality traits that make us a little different from everyone else. Do you know what some of your traits are? What was it about you that made you a little bit (or a lot) different from members of your family?

Each trait is a fundamental building block of personality. These basic inborn traits determine many individual differences in personality. While core traits are present at birth, they're influenced and modified by our environment and how we are reared.

There are numerous personality theories and explanations. One is the Myers-Briggs Type Indicator (MBTI). It provides a practical way to identify, translate, and understand core differences in personality. The MBTI identifies four sets of contrasting personality traits or preferences. Each trait, identified by a single letter, identifies a preference which is the conscious or unconscious choice in a certain designated realm.

Now, you may have heard about this before, or you don't believe in this, but you may find something new here. I'm going to select one mode of personality, expand upon this, and identify your brain's influence. In using this exercise with thousands of individuals, I've seen how understanding this model and the brain's influence has allowed us to discover who we are, make better use of our God-given personalities, and accept the way we were created.

According to type theory, everyone uses all eight of the traits, but one trait out of each pair is preferred and more fully developed. This is similar to the fact that while we have two hands and use both of them, we tend to prefer using one hand to the other. Most people are either right-handed or left-handed. When using your preferred hand, tasks are usually easier, take less time, and are less frustrating—and the end result is usually better. We will focus only on one pairing of traits, the extrovert (E) and the introvert (I).

As I present the various preferences, you'll notice many variations. For example, one extrovert may fit all the characteristics mentioned. In fact, on a scale of 0 to 10, this particular E may be a 10 and would be what we call a Total E, whereas another extrovert may be a 6 on the scale. Some people may find themselves having characteristics of both preferences in each pair. It's normal if a person does not have a strong preference either way.

The MBTI is a tool that doesn't stereotype people or place them in watertight boxes. It's more like a zip code. It tells you the state, city, and neighborhood where you hang out, but not the specific address.

A key aspect of the MBTI is its nonjudgmental nature. The MBTI is grounded in the belief that while different approaches to interacting exist among individuals, no one set of preferences is better or worse than any alternative set of preferences. Thus, the MBTI does not attempt to change behavior to meet a given ideal. Rather, it encourages individuals to understand and appreciate their own and others' personality preferences. Again, it's the brain.

Let's summarize what an E and I are like. You have your own definitions of what an extrovert and an introvert are, but let's be clear about them. These qualities delineate the way people prefer to interact with the environment or the way they are energized.

Extroversion

An extrovert (E) gains energy from people. E's are people oriented. But, an introvert (I) is energized by being alone and is privacy oriented.

The extroversion (E) and introversion (I) preferences focus on how we gain energy. You and I are like batteries. When a battery is attached to a charger, energy flows into the battery. When the battery is powering a lightbulb, energy flows out of the battery.

Energy flows *into* extroverted types when they are around people. Energy flows *out* of extroverted types when they are quietly reflecting on issues. In contrast, energy flows *into* introverted types when they are able to reflect quietly, while energy flows *out* of them when they are interacting with others.

An E is a social creature and gains energy from interactions with other people. They are approachable by friends and strangers alike. Sometimes they tend to dominate a conversation. Invite them to a six-hour party, and they're on cloud nine. At the end of the party, they're wired and ready to go out with friends for coffee at Denny's. They talk with everyone; in fact, they may share too much too soon on a personal level, which may concern an introvert partner.

E's are not the best listeners. For them, listening is harder than talking because they have to give up the limelight. They may also have a tendency to interrupt.

E's have been described as walking mouths. Instead of thinking first, they talk first and really have no idea what they're going to say until they hear themselves talking. They brainstorm out loud for the entire world to hear, and often need to think out loud to come up with the answer. The ideas they come up with aren't set in concrete. They're still working them out, but they let everyone else in on the process. They tend to talk faster and louder and are a bit more animated. E's also prefer a large playing field in life without too many boundaries.

E's typically like noise. They look forward to the interruption of phone calls, and if the phone doesn't ring, they'll start calling people. When they come home, they turn on the TV or their playlist even though they don't actively watch or listen. They like background noise.

In conflict, they talk louder and faster and believe that if they can say just one more thing, everything will be fine.

E's get lonely when their partner isn't there. They look forward to doing things with their partner rather than just sitting around. Judging from the way E's connect with people, you would think they are very secure; but E's have a high need for affirmation and compliments from everyone, especially from significant people. E's may think they've done a good job, but they won't believe it until they hear it from someone else. They may ask for an opinion too. In other words, they *need feedback.*

Introversion

Introverts need to formulate their thoughts in private before they are ready to share. If pressured to give an immediate, quick answer, their minds shut down. They usually respond with, "Let me think about that" or "I'll get back to you on that."

Often, they're seen as shy or reserved. They prefer to share their time with one other person or a few close friends. Usually quiet among strangers, they love privacy and quiet time to themselves. They learn how to concentrate and shut out noise.

Invite an I to a six-hour party, and she would respond, "Six hours! What will I do for six hours? I'd be wiped out!" So the introvert shows up late, talks to selected people one at a time, and leaves early. That is what's comfortable to them. They may not care for the fellowship time in a Sunday school class or church service, either. Why? It's their brain.

I's are good listeners and hate to be interrupted when they talk. When they're in a relationship, they tend to keep their thoughts to themselves and wish their partner would too, if he or she is an E. An I also tends to be cautious when entering a new relationship.

When asked a question, an I usually takes an average of seven seconds before responding. (The problem is, if the other person is an E, that person usually waits about a second and a half before jumping in to give an answer). Our schools are geared to E children. When the teacher asks a question, all the E children raise their hands, even though they don't know the answer yet. They will formulate the answer as they talk out loud. It would level the playing field if the teacher would say to the class, "Here's a question for you. I'd like all of you to think about your answer for 20 seconds, and then I'll tell you when to raise your hands." A statement like that gives equal opportunity to the I's, who wish other people would rehearse their thoughts before speaking.

I's carry on great conversations with themselves, including what the other person said and their own responses. They can do this so realistically that they believe the conversation actually occurred! This creates some interesting interactions!

I's are suspicious of compliments. In turn, they may give them out sparingly.

When I's are married, they can handle the other person's absence fairly well. Usually, they prefer just being with the other person, without a lot of activity and noise, and are more comfortable with a smaller playing field—one they can control. They have clearly defined boundaries, and their motto is "You stay out of my territory, and I'll stay out of yours."

Can an E and an I be compatible...and what about an extreme I or E? You may assume that two E's and two I's would be more compatible because of their similarities. But other aspects of our personalities need to be factored in because they play a part in the compatibility equation. Frankly, any two personality combinations take work to become more compatible.

The very factor that attracted the E and I to each other before marriage can be the major issue of conflict after marriage, as each person's preference will seem more extreme when viewed in daily proximity.

What can two different preference types do to be compatible? They can accept and verbally praise their partner's differences and uniqueness and avoid trying to make the other into a revised edition of their own preferences.

They can praise God for the strengths in each preference, such as the E's ability to connect socially and the I's stability, strength, and depth of thinking.

E's need to remember that I's can be exhausted by superficial socializing. Introverts prefer less-frequent get-togethers with just a few people, particularly with those they feel comfortable being around. An E can help in a large social gathering by *not* introducing his or her I partner to everyone (which makes the I the center of attention an interminable number of times), by *not* talking too loudly, by *not* revealing personal items about their relationship, and by *not* calling on them to pray out loud or asking them a question that requires an immediate response.

When an E wants to talk to an I, it's helpful to approach the I this way: "Here's something I'm interested in knowing. Why don't you think about it and let me know your response?" An introvert will love this. An extrovert could also single out individuals with whom his I partner would be comfortable in one-on-one conversations.

An E may want to ask her I partner to let her know when his battery has been drained and he needs to leave. But I's also need to remember that an E partner thrives on being with people. One solution would be for an I to encourage his or her partner to go to the party before the I does in order to have more time to socialize. Above all, an I needs to give an E partner more compliments than the I thinks is necessary.

One woman I know married into a family of eight (that's right, *eight*!) extreme extroverts. At family get-togethers, she can only last for about an hour. Then she takes a half hour break alone in another room to revitalize. You might think that's ridiculous or rude. No, it's reality—and the only way it can work. The other family members now understand the difference and accept it.

We can't fight the way God created us as unique beings. But we must seek balance as well as meet one another's needs.

When I's hear their E partners brainstorming out loud, they shouldn't assume what they hear is fact. The E is just processing aloud for the whole world to hear. Just ask the E, "Are you brainstorming again?" and you'll probably hear a "yes." On the other hand, it would helpful for E's to announce they are doing this when it occurs. And when an I is thinking about something, it would be helpful to let the E know instead of letting the E feel ignored. It's easy for an E to feel rejected when the I doesn't say anything (even though there's a lot of talking going on inside the I's mind).

Not only does the introverts' and extroverts' blood travel on separate pathways, each pathway requires different neurotransmitters. The pathway extroverts use is activated by dopamine. Dopamine is a powerful neurotransmitter most closely identified with movement, attention, alert states, and learning.

Extroverts have a low sensitivity to dopamine, but they require large amounts of it. How do they get enough? Parts of the brain release some dopamine. But extroverts need its sidekick, adrenaline, which is released from the action of the sympathetic nervous system, to make more dopamine in the brain. So, the more active the extrovert is, the more dopamine is increased. Extroverts feel good when they have places to go and people to see. Do you relate to this or not? Your brain is involved!

Introverts are highly sensitive to dopamine—with too much they feel overstimulated. They use an entirely different neurotransmitter on their more dominant pathway.[2] As one writer puts it,

> Extroverts are alert for sensory and emotional input. When they get stimuli, they can answer quickly because the pathway is rapid and responsive. Their short-term memory is on the tip of their tongue, so while the introvert is still waiting for a word, the extrovert has spit out several. Extroverts need more input to keep their feedback loop working. Their system alerts

the sympathetic nervous system, which is designed to take action without too much thinking.[3]

If we combine the recipe from genetics, messages given by neurotransmitters, brain pathways, and functions of the autonomic nervous centers, what picture emerges? The complete process and feedback loop for each end of the introvert/extrovert continuum.

Researchers discovered that introverts had more blood flowing to their brains than extroverts. This indicates more internal stimulation. Whenever blood flows to an area of your body, that area becomes more sensitive. The other finding was that the blood traveled along different pathways. The researchers found the introverts' pathways were more complicated, involved with the parts of the brain dealing with internal experiences such as remembering, solving problems, and planning. The extroverts' pathways are fast-acting and easily adaptive. Their main pathway is short and less complicated. Their blood flows to the area of the brain controlling visual and auditory sensation. Those involved in these studies conclude that the behavioral differences between the two comes from using different brain pathways.

Let's summarize the introverted process:

Introverts walk around with lots of thoughts and feelings in their heads. They are mulling—comparing old and new experiences. They often have an ongoing dialogue with themselves. Since this is such a familiar experience, they may not realize that *other* minds work in different ways. Some introverts aren't even aware that they think so much, or that they need time for ideas or solutions to "pop" into their heads. They need to reach back into long-term memory to locate information. This requires reflection time without pressure. They also need to give themselves physical space to let their feelings and impressions bubble up. During REM sleep or while dreaming, this pathway integrates daily experiences and stores them in long-term memory, where they are filed in many areas of the brain. Introverts are in a constant distilling process that requires lots of "innergy."[4]

Introversion is at its root a type of temperament. It is not the same as shyness or having a withdrawn personality, and it is not pathological. It is also not something you can change. But you can learn to work *with* it, not *against* it.

The strongest distinguishing characteristic of introverts is their energy source: Introverts draw energy from their *internal world* of ideas, emotions, and impressions. They are energy conservers. They can be easily overstimulated by the external world, experiencing the uncomfortable feeling of "too much." This can feel antsy or in a torpor. In either case, they need to limit their social experiences so they don't get drained. However, introverts need to balance their alone time with outside time, or they can lose other perspectives and connections. Introverted people who balance their energy have perseverance and the ability to think independently, focus deeply, and work creatively.

Introverts are more likely to...

- Keep energy inside, making it difficult for others to know them
- Be absorbed in thought
- Hesitate before speaking
- Avoid crowds and seek quiet
- Lose sight of what others are doing
- Proceed cautiously in meeting people and participate only in selected activities
- Not offer ideas freely; may need to be asked their opinion

- Get agitated without enough time alone or undisturbed

- Reflect and act in a careful way

- Not show much facial expression or reaction[5]

Remember—it's your brain!

Where do you go from here? Where do you go with this information? It could change your relationships. You can thank your brain for being the way you are.

CHAPTER 7

Thanks for the Memories...I Think

Years ago, I read an article about some of our wild animals and their characteristics. One especially took my interest since we had many of these around my home in the hills of Hollywood. It was the coyote. Smaller than the wolf, it is sometimes referred to as the American Jackal. One of the terms used to describe this animal was "the trickster." For some reason, these animals gained this reputation. Coyotes appear in the tales and traditions of Native Americans as a savvy and clever animal, with the ability to fool both other animals as well as humans. I should know—I lost a number of chickens to them! Often, they run in packs and work together to lure their prey so the entire pack can feed.

Well, we have part of our life that is considered a trickster...our memory. Sometimes our memories are accurate, while other times they are distortions. Sometimes you may have difficulty with certain parts of your experiences, and other times it feels like every part of your memory is affected. How do you respond when you struggle with your memories? Most of us are bothered when we can't remember. Some of us also struggle with "intrusive" memories. Those are memories that just show up and stay around—like a song that gets stuck and plays over and over again. When that happens, it's easy to feel like you're losing control or going crazy. You may try to block out those intrusive memories and keep from paying attention to them, but that doesn't work. Between these intrusive memories and the memory gaps, our memories really do play tricks on us.

From time to time, it can be helpful to ask a few simple questions about our memories. Think of this as a routine brain audit.

Do you have difficulty remembering simple things such as names or numbers? Can you learn simple tasks? (This is memory!)

	Yes	No
Some of the time?		
Most of the time?		
Never?		

Do you forget names or places or when you set a date?

	Yes	No
Some of the time?		
Most of the time?		
Never?		

Memory is so important. It ties us to the past but keeps us tied into the present. Most of us will struggle with our memory not being as sharp as it used to be. Part of our problem is not just memory but retrieving the information on demand.

Why are some of us better at memory than others? Well, about half of our memory comes from genetics. Some people are better at memory just naturally. Some of us have to really work at it. Environment makes up the other part. Your environment is what you do and how you treat your body and mind.

How We Remember

All the cues come together, and information is sent to the part of your brain that is associated with sight and sound. Information is sent from one cell to another, and your brain does wonders with what is sent. Like a computer, your memory *stores* information as memories, *retrieves* that information when you need it, and finally, *encodes* the information. Let's examine each of those steps together.

Storage

There are two factors involved in the storage of your memories—short-term and long-term. As you might assume, short-term is information your mind stores for immediate recall, but it usually is limited to small amounts when it comes to the amount stored, and it's usually for a short period of time. What's going on in your brain at this time? Well, your brain is very involved in the creation and storage recall of short-term memories. Your brain is full of neurons which are nerve cells. There is a very active neuron in the front part of your brain where short-term memories are stored. This is an area that produces sight, and it continues to be active after you look at an image. So…the more active your brain is, the more likely you'll be able to both store and retrieve a memory.

Long-term memory can store information for not just a day, but for months and years. Many scientists believe that a memory is formed when a brief pattern of electrical impulses moves through a network of neurons, strengthening connections between the affected brain cells. This leaves a "memory trace" in the brain, which is revived when the information is later recalled. Researchers now know that certain attributes of a memory are grouped with other similar recollections; for example, the smell of roasted peanuts may be grouped together with memories of watching baseball games as a kid. When you recall information, your brain cross-references the many different attributes of that memory. Using techniques like *functional magnetic resonance imaging* (MRI), researchers have been able to map the connectivity between brain regions.

Retrieval

Memories can be retrieved via one of two processes: recall or recognition. Recall involves directly accessing the memory. You also use recall when you remember the name of a movie you saw a week ago. Recognition, on the other hand, uses cues to help you retrieve a memory. When you were in school, you used recognition every time you took a multiple-choice test.

Encoding

What is encoding? When you encode a message, you simply extract the meaning of that memory in a way that makes sense to you. It's conveying data from one form to another. It's the first step in the memory process.

Memory Boosters

If you are concerned about your memory not being as sharp as it used to be, it probably isn't. Welcome to the golden age. Our ability to pay attention does decline with age. Because most seniors accept outdated cultural ideas about "dotty old people," they underestimate their need to practice mental skills, which are particularly high in reasoning and verbal expression, and try to evade intellectual tasks—exactly the opposite of what they should do to stay sharp.

What can you do to boost your memory and to strengthen your brain? The following suggestions may seem a bit strange, but they work, and that's what counts. Your memories and ability to remember can be activated and sharpened. Your ability to remember can be enhanced to the extent that you may be shocked as well as pleasantly pleased.

What is presented here is going to help you enrich your brain. This is how you can enhance your life. Some suggestions will be new, and some may be familiar ones you already use. Are you getting the most out of those you are using?

Don't attempt too much at one time. Don't overload your brain. Just focus on *one memory task* at a time. Remember, this is an idea book to help you get started on beginning the process of helping your brain.

In order to remember more, remember less.

Am I kidding? No. By *remember less,* I mean you should try to remember more of the important items and less of the unimportant. You can't remember everything, nor do you want to. Set up files, keep a weekly and daily calendar, use Post-its (just don't let the dog eat them by counter surfing—yes, that's happened to me!), make lists and put them on the fridge or bulletin board. We live by passwords today. Make them accessible. Make a password file. Use portable files that are handy. I have a list of 30 to 40 names and addresses of key people, and a listing of the four individuals who have my medical records—as well as Power of Attorney and Advance Directive. I also have 15 people listed in my will (who gets what and where it is). I have a list of all banks and accounts.

Keep items in the same place.

Always (no deviations) keep important items in the same safe place—keys, purse, wallet, calendar. Develop a routine—and once again, if you have a dog, be sure to prevent counter surfing. My golden retriever taught me to be more organized. If anything was left out on the counter, she would grab it and chew it up. This included sticky notes, my wallet, and several pens. I've also learned if a pet takes something they shouldn't, it's not the dog's fault. We left it too accessible!

Learn that name.

If I meet you, I will use your name several times in conversation. In my mind, I'll say it again and again and tell myself your name begins with a *T*.

Here are some additional suggestions to help you remember names:

- Whenever you talk to someone, look at them. Look them in the eyes. If you didn't hear them or understand, ask them to repeat. It's better to understand rather than fake it. I know I do better when I hear what was said a second time.

- Do you grasp everything the first time you read it? Probably not. This is how we remember instructions. We all learn in different ways. I'm a visual learner, so I would rather "read" names than "hear" them. If you're a visual learner like I am, you may want to write names down.

- Sometimes I choose a characteristic about a person I've just met. I say it to myself several times, along with their name, and then it's mine!

- If you are trying to remember information, break it down into *small* pieces and repeat it again and again in your mind. If you are given new information, such as a new name, what can you associate it with in order to remember it?

Put your brain to work.

Another way to help protect you from experiencing memory loss is to regularly engage in training exercises that help you practice specific cognitive abilities (such as attention or processing speed). Here are three examples of cognitive exercises that work. Remember: Your brain is a muscle in need of exercise!

- Strengthen your powers of attention by opening a book to a random page and counting the number of words without touching the page. If you lose count, begin again until you finish the page. Strengthen your ability to concentrate by introducing distractions, such as turning on a TV or music.

- Boost information processing speed by examining a photograph you have not seen before for one minute. Then, turn over the photo and jot down as many details from it as you can remember. As your processing speed improves, shorten the time you spend examining each new photo.

- Increase your short-term memory by listening to the Top

10 countdown of popular tunes of your favorite radio sta-
tion, then trying to remember the song titles in order. As
your short-term memory improves, try to remember the
names of the artists, as well.[1]

Meditate mindfully.

I came across a process called *mindfulness meditation*. You may
have heard the term *meditation*, but not *mindfulness*. It's a simple
process:

> This form of meditation involves focusing your aware-
> ness on sensory stimuli in the present moment, while
> ignoring intrusive thoughts and inner chatter. You
> know what I mean—random self-talk for one.
>
> Mindfulness meditation can slow a racing mind, help
> you pay attention to information you need to learn,
> and improve your ability to focus without becom-
> ing distracted and jumping from thought to thought.
> Research suggests it may even help reverse memory
> loss.[2]

Make a weekly plan.

For years, I've followed the principle of making a weekly plan.
By doing this, I don't have to carry my plans in my mind. I do
enjoy checking off item after item. I do keep the list flexible, so
I'm not dominated and controlled by my list. Often, I will run my
list through my mind to see if I can remember it. As I'm driving to
meet with others, I sometimes create a photograph in my mind of
who will be there. Sometimes I surprise myself by either how much
I remember...or how much I don't!

Make your memories stand out.

Keep your memories fresh and make them stand out by using them in a different way. Empower those memories! How? Use some unique elements or associations so that the information stands apart from other information you may be exposed to at the same time.

- Take a snapshot: Create a mental "photograph"—a visual record of what you want to remember. Notice as many details as possible.

- Prepare a speech: Pretend you must describe or explain the information you want to remember to someone else. Rehearsing details—especially out loud—will help fix them in your mind.

- Sing it: Make up a song or jingle containing the information you're trying to remember, such as a shopping list.

- Create a vivid mental image: For example, to help you remember to buy peanut butter, spaghetti, and olives at the supermarket, try picturing yourself with peanut butter smeared in your hair, a necklace of olives, and a hula skirt made of spaghetti strands. The vivid image should make your shopping list easier to recall.[3]

Open a book.

You may find this hard to believe, but if you want to nourish your brain...read. It's one of the best ways to sharpen your brain. When you read, you have more time to think. When you read, you're processing the written material, and this activates the brain and encourages it to work harder and better. The more parts of your brain that get involved, the better it is for your thinking. And what you read makes a difference.

Leisurely reading is all right, but it appears that the more involved you are in the thinking process, the better it is for your brain, since this activates the thinking and decision-making activity.

When it comes to reading, there is one problem that needs to be addressed. Nowadays, more and more of what we read is on a screen. This form of reading is different from the written page. Screen reading does not help the brain to be stimulated. The brain loses its ability to retain information the longer we stare at screens, hindering the process that allows us to read deeply. The solution? Read books and magazines—not the screen.[4] Your brain will appreciate this!

Pick up the pen.

Another way to enrich your brain is journaling. Yes, journaling enriches your brain. But it needs to occur longhand and not on a computer—nor using Facebook or Twitter or whatever is the current rage. Pressing down on the page with a pen or pencil has an impact upon your brain. Journaling drains the brain of its pockets of pain. The more we confront the pain of the past and the present, the less clutter there is in our mind. The more we write, the greater the clarity of our thoughts.

Journaling is no longer old-fashioned. It's something we all need to do—*now*. Journaling does more than just help you record your memories or find self-expression.

What are some of the short- and long-term health benefits of journaling? Here are five benefits of journaling:

1. Journaling reduces stress. An overabundance of stress can be damaging to your physical, mental, and emotional health. One study showed that expressive writing (like journaling) for only 15 to 20 minutes a day three to five times a week over the course of a four-month period

was enough to lower blood pressure and improve liver functionality. In addition, writing about stressful experiences can help you manage them in a healthy way. Journaling can be a pre-bedtime meditation habit to help you unwind and de-stress.

2. Expressive writing can strengthen your immunity and decrease your risk of illness. Those who journal show improved immune system functioning (it strengthens immune cells!) as well as decreased symptoms of asthma and rheumatoid arthritis. Expressive writing has been shown to improve liver and lung function and combat certain diseases; it has even been reported to help the wounded heal faster.

3. Journaling helps keep your brain in functioning shape. It boosts memory and comprehension in a healthy way. It also increases working memory capacity, which may reflect improved cognitive processing.

4. A unique social and behavioral outcome of journaling is this: It can improve your mood and give you a greater sense of overall emotional well-being and happiness. Journal for your brain's sake and your body's sake.

5. Journaling strengthens emotional functions. As journaling habits are developed, benefits become long-term, meaning that diarists become more in tune with their health by connecting with inner needs and desires. Journaling evokes mindfulness and helps writers remain present while keeping perspective. It presents an opportunity for emotional catharsis and helps the brain regulate emotions. It provides a greater sense of confidence and self-identity. Journaling can help

in the management of personal adversity and change
and emphasize important patterns and growth in life.
Research even shows that expressive writing can help
individuals develop more structured, adaptive, and
integrated schemes about themselves, others, and the
world. What's more, journaling unlocks and engages
right-brained creativity, which gives you access to your
full brainpower. Truly, journaling fosters growth.[5]

Journaling is good for you—physically, mentally, and emotionally and is a way to store and keep memories. How do you begin?
Simply start where you are. If you need to initially just write a single
line or detail the specifics of what you had for breakfast, do it. Don't
preoccupy yourself with managing perfect punctuation, grammar,
or spelling. Just write, and don't censor yourself.

Learn a new language.

So, writing is one option. What about adding another language?
There are some amazing facts about being bilingual (or even mul-
tilingual): "The density of gray matter in the brain of bilinguals is
greater than that of monolinguals."[6]

Most of our synapses fire in the gray matter of our brain, and
someone who is bilingual is better at filtering out unnecessary word
clutter. The brain strains to function in two languages, and it is
continually exercising, and this keeps it in shape. A TED Ed video
notes that being bilingual can help a person stave off dementia and
Alzheimer's for up to five years.[7]

Here are a few tips for getting started learning another language:

- Duolingo is an excellent phone app for learning a second
  or third language.

- Google Translate is a user-friendly translation website. You can use it to translate text, speech, and even real-time video. Use this free service to translate words, phrases, and web pages in over 100 languages.

- Watching TV or movies in another language enhances learning. Use subtitles.

- Even if we make mistakes, speaking another person's language honors them and helps grow relationships and expand our worldview.[8]

Whenever you use your hands, you use your brain. The more you think and use your hands, the more your brain is saying thank-you. Whether you play or work with your hands, your brain is stimulated.

Don't try to multitask.

Another thing to consider is multitasking. Can you multitask? No. Can your brain multitask? No. When it comes to paying attention to more than one thing at a time, no. You can do several things at one time, but that doesn't mean you're good at this. You are biologically incapable of multitasking. You are taxing your memory when you try to do several things at once.

This may be a difficult question for you to answer: Is your brain helped more by multitasking or by focused consideration? You may think that in today's fast-paced life, multitasking is the most productive approach to take. It is if you are more productive when you focus on many things at once. But consider: Which way do you actually accomplish the most? When you attempt to multitask, what gets left out?

The more you add to your brain, the less you actually concentrate—and your tendency to make mistakes climbs higher. But here is the main question: What is your brain designed to do? Several things at one time or just one? If you ask too much of this important organ, you may end up with nothing![9]

Spend time with your memories.

As we've touched upon, memory can be very bothersome for many people. Whether it's because you're having difficulty recalling certain aspects of what happened or even having difficulty holding on to new memories, when you can't trust your own mind, you wonder what's next. To add to the complications, many experience intrusive memories and flashbacks (the feeling of reexperiencing events as though they were happening now) that are not only distressing, but can also significantly impact their ability to concentrate or engage in normal daily activities, like work or socializing or praying or sleeping. You can try to gain back a little control by avoiding these memories and pushing them away, of course. Unfortunately, attempts at avoidance often only make the intrusive memories worse.

A key to finding some peace and relief from your troubling memories lies in shifting from *intrusive* rumination to *deliberate* and *reflective* rumination. Your memories are going to come up one way or another. Why fight them? Invite them in. When you try to think critically about what happened to you and your beliefs about it, you give yourself the opportunity to challenge errors in your thinking and eventually grow from the experience.

The best way to do this is to set time aside in your day to do nothing but focus on your thoughts and memories in a purposeful way. By consciously *choosing* to spend time with those thoughts, you'll likely decrease the number of intrusive memories and feel a greater sense of control over your mind. When unwanted thoughts arise at other times during the day, you can remind yourself that you've set aside time to work through these memories and will come back to them in time. You may even choose to briefly document the thoughts and memories as they come up to help inform your later reflection. All these strategies can help you manage your intrusive memories and facilitate your healing and growth.[10]

Get the sleep you need.

Dreams—you have them, and so do I. They have a purpose. Dreams are a vital process for memory consolidation and healing. Memories are consolidated, stabilized, and stored all while you're dreaming. Scientists now recognize the pivotal relationship between periods of rapid eye movement (REM) sleep and dreaming. REM sleep recurs about every 90 minutes in the sleep cycle, totaling about two hours per night on average. REM sleep is unique since many brain regions are *more active* during REM sleep than when we are awake. Sleep studies have found that people awakened from REM sleep report they were dreaming about 80 percent of the time. Dreams also occur during non-REM sleep, but these dreams tend to be briefer and less symbolic—more literal.

Healthy sleep is important since dreams during REM sleep foster emotional restoration. Conversely, disrupted sleep, including insomnia, partial arousals, and nightmares, may contribute to emotional fog.

So, what goes on with our dreams? It appears that what happens during the day is integrated into the deeper portions of our mind, but how? Our current events are linked with similar past experiences. Think of this as a filing system. Your daily events, no matter what, are connected to the system. Different sections of the brain, including the hippocampus and the amygdala, are involved in the work of creating dreams. They also encode emotional memories.

The metaphorical dreams offer opportunities for moments of reflection and insight. One study that was conducted looked at the relationship between dreaming and insight with a mathematical task that could either be solved with lengthy calculations or by sudden insight into a hidden rule. The participants in the study were more than twice as likely to perceive the hidden rule after periods of sleep than after wakefulness. When scientists measured the brain activity of the well-rested participants who perceived the shortcut based on the hidden rule, they observed greater activity in brain regions involved in memory, like the prefrontal cortex.

So, what about you? What is your sleep pattern? Do you remember any of your dreams? Are your dreams relaxing or disturbing? What is your brain doing during this time?

There are probably several different groups of individuals reading this book. Some will give up and say the suggestions don't work. Others will follow the suggestions and discover that change is possible. This latter group is always looking for new ways to "train their brains."

I took classical piano lessons for ten years. In order to memorize various selections, I had to focus upon the piece and play it again and again. I couldn't let my mind wander. I would rehearse several measures and then play the same material again and again, but add new material each time. Eventually, I could play the selection easily. In the same way, you can train your brain not to just hold on to your old memories, but to keep creating new ones.

Remember—the older you are, the greater the chances that your memory is not as sharp as it used to be. Your body ages, and you develop wrinkles, *but changes of the brain are not inevitable.* Take one or two of the suggestions in this chapter and work on sharpening your brain. It's never too late to enhance your mind!

CHAPTER 8

Rehearse, Repeat

Over the past 70 years, I've seen a number of plays and musicals. I watched, listened, and enjoyed myself. The actors and actresses were delightful to observe. The lines they spoke or words they sang seemed to roll off their lips with little or no effort. Their sense of timing was amazing. On one occasion, I went backstage during an intermission and thought I would see the performers resting or consuming food or beverage, but I was surprised to see several practicing their lines again and again and again. Even though they had spent hundreds or thousands of hours practicing, they continued to practice. What I saw when they came on stage to perform was the result of hundreds and thousands of hours.

Why do actors and actresses spend so much time practicing their lines? It's obvious: It's the only way they will learn. This is a must. I learned this principle while attending Westmont College. We had chapel each day, and a speaker shared this with us. (I dislike admitting that I don't remember the name of the speaker.) He said if you will take one chapter from the Bible and read it aloud every day for a month, it will be yours for life. Several of us took him up on this, and we discovered he was right. In a sense, memorizing those words tattooed them on our brains.

We are forgetful creatures. In the course of a single day, we'll forget 70 percent of what happened to us. After several days, about 90 percent of that information will have disappeared.[1] Rehearsing the information you need, reminding yourself of it in bite-sized pieces, will help the retention process. Every time you go over the material, add something new. And review as soon as you can.

How many rehearsals does it take for you to retain? Experiment until you find what works for you. Don't compare your learning ability with others. We're all unique. For me, I have difficulty with names unless I repeat them several times in conversation—and then there's a lock. I go over the pieces of information I need again and again. If I find something that works better—such as a new fingering while playing the piano—I will practice that more.

The rehearsal of information can involve writing what you want to remember, describing it verbally, or teaching it. I have taught graduate school for over 50 years. When I have to transfer what I know to another person, I find that what I share for their benefit has an even greater impact upon my retention. Many teachers retain what they want to learn by rehearsal—they teach their class by teaching it to an empty classroom. And once again, speaking out loud is the best way. Through rehearsal and repetition, you're in the process of tattooing this information on your brain.

Deliberate Practice

I like stories. I like to tell stories. At my age, I can't always count on getting the details correct, so I write them out in minute detail and mentally rehearse them, and my comfort level goes up.

Now let's get practical (and honest). I think we can all use some help in recalling and remembering. These suggestions may seem silly or redundant or repetitive. But give them a try. Your brain needs all the help you can give it. For change to occur, we must practice...and keep practicing. There's that key word: *practice*.

> It's the reason some individuals rise to the top of their profession, when others don't. It's not just a matter of basic raw talent. Consider the findings of Geoff Colvin in the book *Talent Is Overrated*. In looking at outstanding sports figures, as well as musicians, he suggests the difference that accounts for their success over that of their peers is *not* talent, but practice. Even for those with an abundance of natural, above-average talent, talent wasn't enough. What separates the average musician or sports star from the better is just *practice*. Deliberate practice. To rise above, they had to put forth ongoing, consistent practice.[2]

You know what practice is. You've done it, and so have I. It's demanding, and it's not easy. As I've said before, I grew up "practicing piano." For ten years! Some days, I applied myself for an hour, and I improved. Other days, I went through the motions, daydreaming and watching the clock. "Deliberate practice" is the type of practice that is *designed* to improve what it is that you're doing. In most ventures, "designed" means having another person work with you, such as a teacher or coach or mentor or counselor. They can see what you cannot see and can suggest improvements to your practicing.

In his book, Colvin describes it this way:

> Becoming significantly good at almost anything is extremely difficult without the help of a teacher or coach, at least in the early going. Without a clear, unbiased view of the subject's performance, choosing the best practice activity will be impossible; for reasons that may be simply physical (as in sports) or deeply psychological, very few of us can make a clear, honest assessment of our own performance. Even if we could, we could not design the best practice activity for that moment in our development—the type of practice that would put us on the road to achieving at the highest levels—unless we had extensive knowledge of the latest and best methods for developing people in our chosen field. Most of us don't have that knowledge.[3]

Practice positive self-talk

This even applies to changing our self-talk. Whether it's a trusted, insightful friend, a counselor, a spouse, a teacher, or a sponsor, working with someone who can assist you, so you're not working alone, is important. Who do you have in your life that could help you strengthen your brain?

Deliberate practice means identifying what areas need improving. It also means there's a high amount of repetition. In changing your self-talk, it's not enough to identify healthy, realistic thoughts and repeat them once. Because of how deeply entrenched our old, toxic thoughts become, we may need to say the new thoughts hundreds of times before we truly change our thinking for a healthier thought life. (You talk to yourself. I know you do. We all do.)

Changing your self-talk will take time because of the thousands of times the old statements have been expressed. Don't give up! This may sound excessive, but remember: Change is possible. Others have done this with great success—you can too! It will work!

It's important to hear what you're saying to yourself. Listen for negative thoughts, misbeliefs, or toxic, disoriented statements. Pay attention to your self-talk.

Develop a new habit called Self-Talk Awareness (STA). Make an agreement with yourself to become more aware of your inner dialogue.

Develop a reminder system. Place notes to yourself in appropriate places such as the car, bathroom, fridge, purse, or briefcase. Any constant visual reminders will work. On small cards, jot down one or two words, each summarizing your self-talk, such as *distorted* or *not true.*

Keep these with you at all times in your pocket, purse, or briefcase. Seeing this in print will have a greater impact. This is just to make you more aware of how busy your mind is. Evaluate what you've written down. Is it realistic, the truth, positive, constructive? Or is it negative, a misbelief, or toxic?

Let's consider another facet of self-talk. It drifts. And as a drifting boat can get into trouble, so can the mind. Thoughts also wander. Sometimes there's more energy involved in wandering. It can be more active than drifting. We say of a child, "He wandered away," or remark that a husband "wandered from the marriage."

We all have wandering minds. Even when you're focused on a particular subject or speaker or engaged in a personal activity, your mind may wander away from your intended purpose. It's easy to begin daydreaming, planning, fantasizing, or just aimlessly drifting about. Sometimes we can become entangled where we've allowed ourselves to drift: to future events, past painful encounters, worries, and so on.

God understands. Consider this Scripture verse: "The Lord searches all hearts and minds and understands all the wanderings of the thoughts" (1 Chronicles 28:9 AMPC). Your mind has "a mind of its own," so to speak. Regardless of your good intentions to keep it under control and in balance, it still wanders away into thoughts about the past, future, pain, or loss. I might not be aware of all my thoughts, but God certainly is. He "understands all the wanderings of the thoughts."

It's not necessary to stop the wandering. Instead, accept its presence and discover where it takes you. It doesn't help to become angry and frustrated over it. Instead, learn to notice your wandering. As soon as you realize your mind is drifting, just accept it. You don't want to create a battleground for your mind. Fighting your wandering mind may make it wander even more.

It's difficult to slow yourself down to meditate, pray, or even concentrate on reading something (such as this book!). Everyone's mind wanders. So, relax. You're normal. But you can learn to realize more quickly that your mind is wandering. Once that happens, decide whether you want to let it wander, or bring it back to the subject at hand.

As you become aware of your self-talk and how it is affecting your thought life, you will need to become deliberate in changing your thoughts. Deliberate practice involves constant feedback. You need to see that your time and effort is making a difference. As you practice reframing your self-talk in a positive light, take note of the changes in your emotions and behavior.

Deliberate practice will stretch your brainpower. It's hard mental work. You'll be working against what your brain is used to doing, fighting against the direction your brain is used to going. Old patterns of thinking need to be discarded and replaced right away. One way is to write down the thought you want to discard on a piece of paper, then wad it up. Either throw it in the trash or burn it. Think of this—the repetition of positive thoughts about yourself, in place of the old, negative ones—as a rehearsal for living your life in a new and better way.

Imagine that you've just landed a part in a play. It's your big chance. You've dreamed of an opportunity such as this for years. You have two months to rehearse until the play opens. So, what do you do in the meantime? Sit around? Spend more time at your day-time job? Wait until the night before the play opens? Not at all! Your work is just beginning. You need to rehearse! You need to practice! You'll spend hours reading your lines, talking them out, and putting inflection and emotion into them to make them come alive. And can you relax once this happens? Probably not, for you can always refine and improve.

Rehearsals are part of life. Musical groups spend many hours a day in rehearsal before recording a three-minute selection. Sports teams spend weeks in training camps, preparing for the upcoming season, going over their plays again and again. It's the only way for athletes to improve and get in shape. We rehearse presentations for work or job interviews, for classes, for preaching sermons, for more things than we even realize. We even rehearse conversations in our minds—conversations with those who have ignored us, angered us, or hurt us. We run through what happened (with embellishments, of course), and rehearse what we would like to say in future interactions, carefully choosing words that will guarantee we come out on top the next time. Sounds like self-talk, doesn't it?

We rehearse the way we'll face upcoming events that make us feel fearful. We rehearse past experiences, reliving the way they occurred, or reinventing different outcomes of the way we wish they had happened. Most of us spend more time rehearsing than we realize. And sometimes, we create scenarios and interactions that are far from what actually occurred. Our new version of the outcome becomes very real to us—we believe they're real because we've rehearsed them again and again.[4]

Don't expect practice to be enjoyable or fun. It's work. You will have to put intentional effort into what you are doing. Sometimes, you may question the work's effectiveness. But keep your long-term goal in sight. Changes may be slow, but you will see them!

Most of us not only have to practice in order to learn, we need to review again and again. As an actor learns his lines for a play or a film, he goes over them again and again. That allows them to go from being words on a page to becoming part of him. They take on a life of their own. It's the same with the new phrases you're speaking to yourself. They need to become part of your life, and you need to repeat them. The first time you go over one in your mind, it may feel awkward. You may not feel like it's "really you" yet. But the more you practice your new responses, the more they become the new you.

Mental Pictures

We want to make our brain function at its best. How can you help your brain be all it can be? How can it function so you get the most from its potential? Let's spend some time focusing on helping your brain remember. There are four simple suggestions which, if applied, will make a difference.

The mind's eye

The first is visualization, or seeing with your "mind's eye" what it is you're trying to remember. Whatever you are trying to remember, see it in your mind. Picture it. Paint a mental picture, which uses all our faculties.

The more unusual the picture, the more unforgettable it will be. Go back to the picture you created and visualize it in a "weird" way. That weirdness will stick out to you, helping you remember your information because of its unique associations.

Location

The next procedure is often called the method of *location*. This could be where you are or where you need to be. We live by routine, and yet we're often not conscious of where we are or need to be. Instead of doing everything by rote or routine, describe your process verbally. Tell another person the steps you take to go somewhere, or write it out from memory. You may be surprised by what you remember (or don't). You may want (in order to make your brain work harder) to change some of your patterns or routines. You can expand or diminish your routine, but be sure to describe what you are doing. List-making is a part of our life, but too often it's automatic. Let your brain become aware of your own list to make your list more productive.

Names and faces

What about names and faces? Do they come easily, or do you struggle? We all have times when names or faces are elusive, and we need to "fake it" to get through a conversation. I call this the "I'll never forget old what's his name" syndrome.

If this memory lapse is causing difficulty in your life, enlist your brain to help. I know some who pray for the ability to remember. You can also take care to make associations with a person's name or face when you see them. Ask yourself what's unique about that person's face or hairstyle. You can also try associating their looks with something else (but be careful you don't tell them!).

No matter which method you try, remember the principle of repetition. When I meet someone, I try to say their name out loud at least three times during the conversation and several times silently. I tell my brain, "Carve out a hole to remember Ted."

Chunking

Chunking is an activity we all engage in at one time or another. It's simply a matter of breaking a string of numbers into smaller and more manageable units (or chunks). By doing this again and again, your brain makes a habit of remembering.

Here are some practical, simple suggestions for "chunking" that engage your brain and help you function better. These are suggestions in the book *Age-Proof Your Mind* by Zaldy Tan:[5]

1. Select a picture from a magazine. Close it and write down as many details as you can remember. Look at it again and write down those items you missed. Do this every day for a week. You may be surprised at your improvement.

2. Select a TV show and select ten questions to answer about this program. After watching it, answer your questions. These could include names of the cast, color of clothing, types of clothing, time of day for the settings, etc.

3. Select four individuals you saw today and describe how they were dressed. Be as detailed as you can.

4. Have someone read a story to you and then tell it in your words and with as much detail as you can.

5. Have someone read each set of numbers to you aloud, pausing one second between each digit. Repeat the numbers in the correct order.

6-7

2-9-7

4-2-9-3

8-9-3-6-4

2-8-1-7-6-5

8-1-7-2-4-6-5

6-3-9-8-2-5-1-4[6]

6. Have someone read you the following list of unrelated words, allowing for a one-second pause in between words. Then try to recall as many words as you can from the list. They don't have to be in any particular order.

Bracelet

Hammer

Violet

Truck

Jelly

Dairy

Chin

Atlas

Teapot

Clarinet[7]

There are many other resources which can be used to test your memory and strengthen your ability to concentrate and focus.

We all would like to dodge the memory changes of aging, but we know that the older we get, the more our brains shrink. From age 20 to 40, the brain remains fairly stable. But time brings changes. By late middle age, we lose an average of about one percent of our brain cells every year (and you're how old?). Between the ages of 18 and 95 you lose nearly 50 percent of your brain cells. The lost tissue is replaced by fluid and dead space. We have large, dark holes in our skull. Some people lose more brain cells than others. But all of this is normal aging.[8] It does not mean we can't be sharp in our older age.

Now that we've taken a tour through the brain and looked at some activities to help keep it fit, it's time to look at some specific issues many of us will navigate as we get to know our brains.

PART TWO

CHAPTER 9

Worry on the Mind

The word *worry* comes from an Anglo-Saxon root meaning "to strangle" or "to choke." When you experience anxiety, your body responds. Usually, your muscles tighten and your heart races. Worry has been defined as the *thinking* part of anxiety, as a series of thoughts and images that are full of emotion—all negative. These thoughts are rarely uncontrollable, but they focus on an event that has an uncertain outcome. The worrier is convinced beyond a shadow of a doubt that the outcome will be negative.

There are many ways to understand or describe worry. Here are just a few:

- Worry is thinking turned into poisoned thoughts.

- Worry is a small trickle of fear that meanders through the mind until it cuts a channel into which all other thoughts are drained.

- A church billboard in Colorado described worry as "a darkroom where negatives develop."

- Worrying about something is like having a brain cramp that won't let go of your worry. The more you worry, the more you cut a groove in your brain, and the more worry finds a home in which to reside.

- Worry is like an invading army that creeps ashore at night and eventually controls the country.

Worry is actually a kind of fear—a special kind. To create it, we elongate fear with two things: anticipation and memory. We then infuse it with our imagination and feed it with emotion. And then we have our creation.[1] And our brain wraps its arms around it.

There are many diseases in our world today, but worry is an old one—a disease of the imagination. It's like a virus that slowly and subtly takes over and dominates our life. When that happens, our ability to live the way we want to is diminished. A Swedish proverb says, "Worry gives a small thing a big shadow."

Many Scripture verses describe the effects of worry and anxiety. And many other verses reveal that a worry-free life reaps many positive rewards. Notice the contrast in the verses that follow:

- Anxiety weighs down the heart, but a kind word cheers it up (Proverbs 12:25).

- A heart at peace gives life to the body, but envy rots the bones (Proverbs 14:30).

- A happy heart makes the face cheerful, but heartache crushes the spirit (Proverbs 15:13).

- All the days of the oppressed are wretched, but the cheerful heart has a continual feast (Proverbs 15:15).

- A cheerful heart is good medicine, but a crushed spirit dries up the bones (Proverbs 17:22).

- Let the message of Christ dwell among you richly as you teach and admonish one another with all wisdom through psalms, hymns, and songs from the Spirit, singing to God with gratitude in your hearts (Colossians 3:16).

Notice what we're commanded to do with the message of Christ—let it *dwell*. Who or what do you dwell on in your mind? When your mind *dwells* on everything that could go wrong, your biochemistry is affected, leading to an adrenaline response. This adrenaline rush can make you prone to even greater anxiety!

This biochemical response is *not* a malfunction of the central nervous system; it is a completely normal response. If a man wearing a ski mask were to burst into your home, your body would immediately respond by registering *trouble*. Adrenaline and cortisol would start racing through your body. But when those hormones are triggered by worry, absent a clear danger signal, they can wreak havoc on your mind and body.

Perhaps you've seen films of the inside of a cockpit of a fighter plane. Most of our military planes rely upon missiles for their weaponry. In front of the pilot is a screen that shows the enemy plane. The pilot guides his or her plane in order to line it up for the missile. When the fighter is correctly lined up, the screen lights up with a "missile lock" message. The missile is locked onto that enemy plane until it's destroyed.

In the same way, worry seems to lock onto a problem and won't let go. Then it sends an alarm signal to the front part of the brain, which analyzes the worry. The front portion sends a signal back to the worry, which says, "Worry now!" The worry then becomes alarmed even more and sends a signal back to the front, and thus it goes on and on. It's like a circuit that can't be broken. It's as though the worry has taken control of the brain and shut out the rest of life around you.

Professional Worrying

When worry invades a person's mind, it can send the brain into a kind of spasm. It's like a lock that is unable to relax and accept anything that is good or positive. All it sees is the negative. And it's not just a fleeting thought, but something that seems encased in cement.

Have you ever had a muscle in a cramp, and you can't get rid of it? One author describes it this way:

> The mind of the worrier, in an effort to anticipate danger or stave off some bad outcome, has gone into a spasm, a lock that can't relax and accept good news. The mind can't let go of the matter at hand and can't see it in any but a negative way. Hours, whole days, weeks, or even years can be poisoned by ruminating on a single fear, one predominating worry.[2]

But here's the good news: Even if you've been a worrier for many years, even if your brain seems to be in a permanent worry cramp, worry is a spasm which can be reversed. I've worked with many (what I call) *professional worriers*. They are good at this. They should be—they've been practicing for years. They've trained their brain to worry. In the same way, they can train their brain to respond in a healthy way.

We train our muscles to play a certain sport, and after a time, we develop "muscle memory." The movements become natural and automatic, and they hardly require our conscious thought. In the same way, we can train the muscle memory in our brains.

Notice Your Thoughts

The phrase *mental noise* describes the thoughts, urges, compulsions, fears, and especially worries that form a constant background noise in our brains. We can give in to the "mental noises" and allow them to dominate our thought life, which slows the functioning of our brain. What we think about (obsessively) can change our brain chemistry, and this can go either way—positive or negative.

A number of the messages we send to ourselves are of little or no value. They limit us. The first step in stopping these messages, of course, is to identify them. Take each thought or worry or fear and evaluate it on a scale from 0 to 10 to clarify its value to your life. When this occurs and you discover the negative effect your thoughts have upon you, the value of these thoughts diminish. You can learn to tell these thoughts, "You are senseless, and I value my brain more than this thought. I'm only going to listen to thoughts that will benefit my brain and not tear it down."[3]

When these troublesome thoughts pop into your brain, you can learn to evaluate them instead of accepting them at face value. Scripture tells us, "We demolish arguments and every pretension that sets itself up against the knowledge of God, and we take captive every thought to make it obedient to Christ" (2 Corinthians 10:5). Sometimes what comes from our brain is true and healthy, and these thoughts energize us. Some of what we hear and receive is just mental noise or false signals.[4] If we challenge what we receive and confront it, consciously determining whether the message is true or helpful, we can change our brain chemistry.

What If Everything Turns Out Fine?

Anxiety thrives on imaginary problems. If you take each harmful "What if..." and phrase it in a positive way, solutions begin to emerge—especially if the answer is within the Scriptures.

Use your imagination. Just imagine positive outcomes. This may go counter to what your mind or brain is telling you. But it's scriptural, and it works. Here are some examples of positive "What if..." thoughts:

Negative: *What if I never get over my worry?*

Positive: *What if I do overcome my worry?*

Negative: *What if I forget what I'm supposed to say?*

Positive: *What if I remember everything I want to say?*

Negative: *What if I mess up and lose my job?*

Positive: *What if I do everything right and keep my job?*

Negative: *What if I never get off my medication?*

Positive: *What if I get off my medication?*

Negative: *What if the new people don't like me?*

Positive: *What if the new people really like me?*

Negative: *What if I fail the test?*

Positive: *What if I pass the test and do very well?*

What are some negatives that you struggle with? How could you turn them into positives?

Go Fast

Learn to identify your worries when they first grip your mind. There is a window of opportunity—it may last less than a minute—during which you can sever the grip the toxic worry has on you before it's too late. For most people, once it gets settled in, the toxicity of the worry lasts for hours, even days or weeks. To cut it off immediately, you must take action.

Deliberately change your actions. Take a walk, talk to your spouse or a friend about something unrelated to your worries, or sing your favorite song loudly. You could write a letter to a friend with whom you haven't communicated in a while. You could get down on your knees and pray. Splash water on your face—or even better, take a cold shower. The old-fashioned remedy of a run around the block followed by a cold shower is still one of the best.[5]

Go Slow

If worries have already taken hold, slow yourself down. Breathe in slowly, and hold your breath for four or five seconds. You can do this whether you're at home or at the mall. Do this several times, and you'll discover that you are more relaxed as well as thinking or moving at a different pace. When you hold your breath, your focus is no longer on the alarm or the pain or whatever has triggered your anxiety. Your breath is helping you relax.

As you continue to breathe in and out, begin to repeat the following Scripture verses:

- You will keep in perfect peace those whose minds are steadfast, because they trust in you (Isaiah 26:3).

- Be made new in the attitude of your minds (Ephesians 4:23).

- Do not conform to the pattern of this world, but be transformed by the renewing of your mind. Then you will be able to test and approve what God's will is—his good, pleasing and perfect will (Romans 12:2).

- With minds that are alert and fully sober, set your hope on the grace to be brought to you when Jesus Christ is revealed at his coming (1 Peter 1:13).

Schedule Your Worry

You and I are creatures of habit. We're comfortable with the routine in our life. And there is nothing wrong with that. And I'm not suggesting that you change your habits and routines. But why not add something new for your brain's sake?

Let me suggest one method of breaking the pattern by taking you into my counseling office. I was working with a man who had a roaring tendency to worry. We had talked through the reasons for his worry, and he had tried some of my suggestions for conquering his problem. But it seemed to me he was resistant to giving up his worry. (This isn't unusual. Many people have worried so long that they have grown comfortable with their negative patterns of thinking. It's actually all they know. They're successful with it and are unsure they will be successful with the new style of thinking.)

So, one day I gave him an assignment that really caught him off guard: "It appears that worry is an integral part of your life," I said, "and you are determined to keep this tendency. But you only worry periodically throughout the day, with no real plan for worrying. So let's set up a definite worry time for you each day instead of spreading it out.

"Tomorrow when you begin to worry about something, instead of worrying at that moment, write down what you're worried about on an index card. Keep the card in your pocket. Each time a worry pops up, write it on the card, but don't worry about it yet. Then, about 4:00 p.m., go into a room where you can be alone. Sit down, take out the card, and worry about the items as intensely as you can for 30 minutes. Start the next day with a new blank card and do the same thing. What do you think about that idea?"

He stared at me in silence for several moments. "That's got to be one of the dumbest suggestions I've ever heard," he finally answered. "I can't believe I'm paying you to hear advice like that."

I smiled and said, "Is it really much different from what you're already doing? Your behavior tells me you like to worry, so I'm just suggesting you put it into a different time frame." As he thought about my comment, he realized I was right: He really wanted to worry. And until he decided he didn't want to worry, there was nothing I could do to help him.

This is very important: *Unless you make a value judgment on your negative behavior, your behavior will never change.* The issue parallels the question Jesus asked the lame man at the pool of Bethesda: "Do you want to get well?" (John 5:6).

You must make some conscious, honest decisions about your fear or worry. Do you like it or dislike it? Is it to your advantage or disadvantage? Is your life better with it or without it? If you're not sure, apply the techniques in this chapter and commit yourself to not worrying for a period of just two weeks. Then, from your own experience, decide whether you prefer a life of worrying or a life of freedom from worry.

Tell Yourself to STOP

During one session of a Sunday school class I was teaching on the subject of worry, I asked the participants to report on an exercise I had suggested the previous week for kicking the worry out of their lives. One woman said she began the experiment Monday morning, and by Friday she felt the worry pattern that had plagued her for years was finally broken.

What accomplished this radical improvement? It was a simple method of applying God's Word to her life in a new way. I have shared this method with hundreds of people in my counseling office and with thousands in classes and seminars.

Take a blank index card, and on one side write the word *STOP* in large, bold letters. On the other side, write the complete text of Philippians 4:6-9:

> Do not be anxious about anything, but in every situation, by prayer and petition, with thanksgiving, present your requests to God. And the peace of God, which transcends all understanding, will guard your hearts and your minds in Christ Jesus. Finally, brothers and sisters, whatever is true, whatever is noble, whatever is right, whatever is pure, whatever is lovely, whatever is admirable—if anything is excellent or praiseworthy— think about such things. Whatever you have learned or received or heard from me, or seen in me—put it into practice. And the God of peace will be with you.

Keep the card with you at all times. Whenever you're alone and begin to worry, take the card out, hold the *STOP* side in front of you, and say aloud, "Stop!" Then turn the card over and read the Scripture passage aloud twice with emphasis.

Taking the card out interrupts your thought pattern of fear and worry. Saying "Stop!" further breaks your automatic habit pattern of worry. Then, reading the Word of God aloud becomes the positive substitute for worry. If you are in a group of people and begin to worry, follow the same procedure, only do it silently.

The woman who shared her experience with the class said that on the first day of her experiment, she took the card out 20 times during the day. But on Friday, she only took it out three times. She said, "For the first time in my life, I have hope that my worrisome thinking can be chased out of my life."

Freedom from worry is possible! It requires that you practice the diligent application of God's Word in your life. This means repetitive behavior. If you fail the first time, don't give up. You may have practiced fear and worry for many years, and now you need to practice consistently the application of Scripture over a long period in order to completely establish a new, fear- and worry-free pattern.[6]

> Worry is an option, not an assignment. God can lead you into a worry-free world. Be quick to pray. Focus less on the problems ahead and more on the victories behind. Do your part, and God will do his. He will guard your heart with his peace...a peace that passes understanding.[7]

Brain Freeze

There it was again. It didn't occur suddenly. It was slight...just enough to know it was there hiding, like something ominous, ready to evolve and dominate whatever you were doing. You knew what was coming, for you've felt it before. Unfortunately, when it comes, sometimes it feels like a cascading onslaught of giant ice cubes.

Once it starts, no amount of rubbing or blinking or shaking of your head can break its entrance or its duration. You've felt it before. It has a name—it's called *brain freeze*. And you know why it occurred, don't you? We all know how to prevent its dominating presence. If only you hadn't inhaled that iced solution.

I remember walking by Baskin Robbins Ice Cream and saw a man with his hand over his head, eyes shut, a grimace on his face, with his teeth clenched shut as tight as possible. He's hoping beyond hope he can stop the progression of this pain (which won't happen). He was the victim of a brain freeze.

Many of us live as though we have a permanently frozen brain. That's a disorder that has a name. Most people have heard of Obsessive Compulsive Disorder, or OCD. The diagnostic term makes the condition sound even stranger than it actually is. In fact, most of us have experienced the symptoms associated with OCD at one time or another. OCD is an amplification of the fears and superstitions most people live with in mild forms all the time. Everyone must deal with surprising, sometimes terrifying and unwanted thoughts now and then. For example, most people have imagined jumping off a tall building, for no apparent reason, while they were standing on the top floor, or imagined defiling a beautiful painting while they were looking at it, even if they liked the painting and had no desire to deface it, or they have been horrified by an image they would like to forget of the death of a loved one that pops into their minds unexpectedly. Once in a great while this kind of intrusive thought or image bothers just about everyone. But if these thoughts recur often and seem uncontrollable or deeply upsetting, then we may be in the domain of OCD.[8]

Usually, however, the symptoms are not that extreme or bizarre. A very common symptom in OCD, for example, is checking. The sufferer must return to his house, office, or car over and over again to *make sure* he did not forget something or leave some switch on that should have been turned off. He will have to check many times before he can finally leave. He checks his briefcase repeatedly before shutting it and checks to make sure he has his wallet hundreds of times a day. He will go online to check his bank balance three to four times in an hour. While waiting in his doctor's office, he checks outside several times to make sure his car hasn't been stolen, and he asks his boss to repeat the assignment he's just been given four times to make sure he heard it right. He also checks in his rearview mirror so often that he's dangerously unaware of what's in front of him. Any one of these types of checking, taken by itself, is not a great concern. But taken as a total package, this disorder becomes a huge obstacle.

OCD starts with the mind not being able to let go of a certain fear. The disordered mind then makes up some magical ritual that needs to be performed to counter the fear. These rituals could include counting or drumming fingers in a certain pattern, starting the morning and ending the evening with everything lined up symmetrically on the desk, or singing a favorite song three times, each a desperate attempt to control the irrational fear. As this pattern sets in, actual physical changes can occur in the brain. Differences have been noted in the brain scans of individuals with OCD, and we have seen these changes resolve after treatment, which is pervasive evidence that this condition is not under voluntary or even unconscious control but is rather a medical problem.

Obsessions are intrusive, unwelcome, distressing thoughts or mental images. It's as though something is tattooed upon our brain. This has the potential for good or bad, depending on what it is. I like the origin for the word *obsess*. It comes from the Latin and it means "to besiege." You feel that your thoughts are plaguing you. Obsessive thoughts are those which seem as though they are tethered to your brain. As soon as you think they're under control, they hop back into your mind with a renewed intensity. These are thoughts which are not healthy nor beneficial. They don't build up, but tear down.

There is another word that we need to recognize: *compulsion*. Compulsions are behaviors rather than thoughts. They come into being in our attempt to get rid of those troublesome thoughts. You may be aware of how absurd some of these are, but it doesn't make any difference. They may bring some relief, but not for long. Remember that we talked about neuroplasticity—changing pathways in the brain, and especially with plaguing thoughts and repetitive behavior.

But the good news is that there are effective treatments for worrying and OCD, and with these treatments, the brain can always change back.[9] First, you train yourself to identify what's real and what isn't. Second, you understand that those thoughts and urges are merely mental noise, false signals being sent from your brain. Third, you learn to respond to those false signals by refocusing your attention on more constructive behavior to the best of your ability at that moment. This is where the hardest work is done and where the change in brain chemistry takes place.[10]

Born Worriers

While some people are born with confidence, others are born insecure. While some people are born calm, others are born wired. While some people are born pushing ahead, others are born holding back. You may be born with a specific characteristic, or you may be vulnerable to develop it later on, in the face of the pressure life usually produces.[11]

The physical perspective on worry helps explain why some people react so strongly when a particular kind of crisis hits, and there are others who do not react at all. We cannot lay all the causation at the feet of those who raised us or life experience. Worries seem to inherit a neurological vulnerability that life events can trigger.

But remember this promise: Destructive worry thinking can be eliminated. The toxic pattern of frenzied worrying can be relearned.[12] Our brains are somewhat plastic, so whatever is going on in those brains can be altered. If our brains can be changed in a negative way, they can be changed in a positive way as well.

CHAPTER 10

The Grieving Brain

*G*rief. It shapes all of your life and the way your entire body functions. The closer you are to the one whom you've lost, the more your body is affected. The physical is impacted, but so is your thinking, such as memory (where did it go?), confusion (your thinking feels like mush), and attention span (it flies away). You are not who you were—and you won't be who you used to be. I know. I've walked the path of grief, and I'm still there. Since 2007, I've lost my wife of 48 years, my 53-year-old daughter (my son died in 1990), my older brother, and my son-in-law, as well as several friends. My body and my mind are not the same.

The passage of grief will take longer than one could ever imagine. It tends to intensify three months after the loss, on special dates, and on the one-year anniversary.[1] But that's just the beginning.

On a current TV show, grief was described like this by a police officer:

> Grief is grief. It's a hole that can't be filled but over time it will shrink enough so that you won't fall in every time you take a step. If there's one thing you can use to make you a better cop, it will be her life, not her death.[2]

Grief takes on many faces, such as disruption, holes, confusion. It disrupts one's entire life. Grief comes from within and doesn't leave one particle of life untouched. It's all consuming. Food doesn't taste the same, nor will the fragrance of a favorite flower be as intense. The frequency of tears clouds vision. Some experience a tightness in their throat or chest, an empty feeling in their stomach, shortness of breath, or rapid heart rate. Eating and sleeping patterns change. Some people sleep and sleep, while others wish that sleep would come. This disruption will decrease in time, but recovery is not a smooth, straightforward path; it's a forward-backward dance.

Prior to the death of a loved one, life was going in a well-established direction. You were someone's parent, spouse, sibling, friend. But the person who died has taken part of your identity with them. That space will always remain in your heart and memory, but the loss of a person you loved has left a hole in your life.[3] Your identity is changing. Eventually, you'll start to take steps into a new identity, but that's a long process—and not one that can be rushed.

It is not just the loss of the loved one that is so painful. It is also all the other losses that occur alongside the one who has died: the way they lived their life, loved, slept, ate, worked, and worshiped are all affected. Often, the death of the loved one brings up not just grief for what has been lost but also for what they never had and what they never will have.

There are behavior changes. Many people say, "I'm just not myself." That's true. They won't be for some time.

Whether the death was expected or sudden, we may experience numbness. The more unexpected and traumatic the loss, the more intense the numbness will be. In some ways, our brain shuts down.

There will be a time when feelings could be described as a time of suffering and disorganization, or even chaos. The trance is over. We talk about scenes rather than stages, for stages vary depending on whom you read. And there are those who bypass some scenes. After the numbness wears off, the pain of separation comes.

One of the clusters of feelings to emerge will be a sense of emptiness, loneliness, and isolation, even when others are next to the person in grief.

The second common cluster of feelings is fear and anxiety. And the fears accumulate. They may come and go or be a constant sense of dread.

Your sleep will be impacted, which impacts your brain. We need our sleep to restore our body as well as our mind. Grief rearranges your sleep, and your sleep rearranges the functioning of your brain.

You may find yourself looking at the pages of a book, but your brain can't handle what you're seeing. I know that my mind plays tricks on me. Sometimes it feels as though you've lost your mind. Your brain doesn't work like it did. Crazy? You're not. It just feels that way. Your mind and your brain feel rearranged. You probably have to use reminders in order to function.

In grief, your brain has to codify and collate an impossible new reality into itself. The data presented doesn't make any logical sense. There has never been anything like this event, so there is no way to connect or relate it to anything else. It doesn't fit. The brain cannot *make* this new reality fit. Like your heart, your brain resists this loss—it can't possibly be true.[4]

Many struggle with their thinking and what they can do. Megan Devine, the author of *It's OK That You're NOT OK*, puts it this way:

> There's a reason you can't get as much done as you used to.
>
> Think of it like this: "Let's say you have one hundred units of brain power for each day. Right now, the enormity of grief, trauma, sadness, missing, loneness, takes up ninety-nine of those energy units. That remaining one unit is what you have for the mundane and ordinary skills of life. That one remaining circuit is responsible for organizing carpools and funeral details. It's got to keep you breathing, keep your heart beating, and access your cognitive, social and relational skills. Remembering that cooking utensils belong in the drawer, not the freezer, that your keys are under the bathroom sink where you left them when you ran out of toilet paper—these things are just not high on the brain's priority list.
>
> Of course, you're exhausted. Your mind, like the rest of you, is doing the best it can to function and survive under very severe circumstances. Please try not to judge your current accomplishments based on what you used to be able to do. You are not that person right now.[5]

There are several ways that grievers attempt to resist the pain. Some fight the pain through denial. They say, "No, it isn't true," or attempt to live their lives as though nothing has happened.

Grieving moves through several levels of denial. Each stage that brings home the reality of the loss is a bit deeper and more painful. A stage is accepting it in our heads, then in our feelings, and finally, when we adjust to life's pattern, to reflect the reality of what has occurred. Your body is involved in all of this.

Grieving is also a disorderly process. It can't be controlled, nor can it be scheduled. Grief will take the shape of a spiral figure rather than a linear one. Grief is not a straight line moving forward only to return the person to where he/she used to be. Someone may think they've left behind that intense pain, and the relief is so refreshing, but the pain is rediscovered again and again. Our mind has difficulty coping with all this.

Grievers may find themselves easily distracted and perhaps disoriented, even if they are usually decisive. Now they may be afraid to make choices. Many find that their sense of time is distorted. Time goes too fast or too slow. Past and future collapse together. A clock can be sitting in front of their face, but it doesn't register. Why does this occur? It's like your brain turned to mush. It's not functioning as well. Its functioning is disrupted.

To assist others with their journey of grief, we need to truly understand the world of grief. This may be uncomfortable for you. Grief is one of the most uncomfortable places to ever live. It hurts, confuses, upsets, and frightens those who are living with it. Perhaps you've been there, but perhaps not. To effectively help someone going through grief, we must enter into this difficult world.

Whenever there is a loss, there will be grief. But some people make a choice not to express all the feelings inside, so their grief accumulates. Saving it up won't lessen the pain; it will only intensify it. Silence covers a wound before the cleansing has occurred. The result will be an emotional infection.

How We Grieve

Is the brain involved in the grieving process? Very definitely. There are two distinct major patterns of grief. These have been given names: intuitive and instrumental. Each one has distinct characteristics. You might experience one of these patterns in your own grieving, or you might follow a blend of the two patterns.

If you're an intuitive griever, you may experience grief as a sense of waves of acutely painful feelings. Intuitive grievers often find themselves without energy and motivation. Their expressions of grief truly mirror their inner experiences. Anguish and tears are almost constant companions. Your grief patterns might look like this:

1. Feelings are intensely experienced.

2. Expressions such as crying and lamenting are a window to the heart of a person's inner experience.

3. Successful adaptive strategies facilitate the experience and expression of feelings.

4. There are prolonged periods of confusion, inability to concentrate, disorganization, and disorientation. This often impairs the ability to complete tasks.

5. Physical exhaustion and anxiety may result.

Because openly expressing and sharing feelings is traditionally identified as a female brain, intuitive grieving is usually associated with women. Of course, this is not always the case; male intuitive grievers grieve in similar ways to female grievers.[6]

If you're an instrumental griever, your grieving process will look a little different. You prefer a problem-solving approach, but your normal problem-solving methods aren't functioning the way they used to. You struggle to talk about or describe what you're feeling.

1. Thinking is predominant to feeling as an experience; feelings are less intense.

2. There is general reluctance to talk about feelings.

3. Mastery of oneself and the environment are most important.

4. Problem-solving as a strategy enables mastery of feelings and control of the environment.

5. Brief periods of cognitive dysfunction are common.

6. Energy levels are enhanced, but symptoms of general arousal go unnoticed.

Intuitive grievers put their energy and expression into their feelings and much less into the cognitive or thinking arena. Grief for the intuitive individual is made up of feelings—painful feelings—and the expression of these is usually through crying.

Instrumental grievers take the energy from grief and go into the thinking arena rather than feelings. It's more of an intellectual experience. This person looks for activities to deal with what he or she is experiencing.[7]

It's rare to find a person who is purely intuitive or purely instrumental. Most people are a mixture of both. They express their grief in a way that reflects both patterns but tends to go toward one end of the continuum or the other.

Traumatic Grief

Some grief is called traumatic grief. Traumatic grief lengthens and multiplies every aspect of the grief process. Traumatic grief is a direct response to disastrous events that threaten safety, security, and beliefs around which we structure and order our lives.

Certain events are more likely to precipitate traumatic grief reactions and share some common themes. Here is a list of descriptors that identify what can bring on traumatic grief reactions:

- Unexpected—The surprise elements stun and shock. We feel dazed and disoriented.

- Uncontrollable—The event is beyond our abilities to change it. We feel powerless and vulnerable.

- Unimaginable—The horrific elements are not familiar to our way of life. Our frame of reference does not include what we are witnessing. We feel appalled and horrified.

- Unfair—We feel like victims who have done nothing to deserve this tragedy. We feel hurt, puzzled, angry, or fearful.

- Unforgivable—We need to blame someone or something. What do we do with our anger, rage, and urge to punish? We feel powerless.

- Unprecedented—Nothing like this has happened before. We don't have a script to follow. We feel directionless.

- Unprepared—We haven't perceived a reason to ready ourselves for an unimaginable catastrophe. Our defense mechanisms may be inadequate to handle the demand. We feel overwhelmed.

No wonder this is overwhelming. Experiencing traumatic loss—witnessing the suffering and death of loved ones—is harrowing. We were not called to experience this.

When death occurs from sudden, unexpected circumstances—such as accident, suicide, or murder—grief reactions are more severe, exaggerated, and complicated. The mourner's capacity to use positive coping mechanisms is overwhelmed.

If you've experienced a traumatic loss, you may be struggling with the issue of unfinished business between you and the one who died. Many people have said they felt like they were dangling with statements unsaid, issues unresolved, and no closure. The person may be gone, but the issues remain, and they're the only one left to try to resolve them. Whatever is unfinished can be a barrier to moving along the path to recovery.

Perhaps our unfinished business is clinging to hurts and offenses from the one who died. Some carry videotapes full of pain in their memory. We carry the offenses of the other person in our mind as a burden. We inflict inner torment upon ourselves. There's a solution. Forgive the person. When we release them, we're released. If we don't forgive, we sentence ourselves to the prison of resentment. Lewis Smedes said it well:

> When you forgive someone for hurting you, you perform spiritual surgery inside your soul; you cut away the wrong that was done to you so that you can see your "enemy" through the magic eyes that can heal your soul. Detach that person from the hurt and let it go, the way children open their hands and let a trapped butterfly go free.
>
> Then invite that person back into your mind, fresh, as if a piece of history between you had been erased, its grip on your memory broken. Reverse the seemingly irreversible flow of pain within you.[8]

We are able to forgive because God has forgiven us. He has given us a beautiful model of forgiveness. Allowing God's forgiveness to permeate our lives and renew us is the first step toward wholeness.

CHAPTER 11

When It Hurts Too Much

The brain is actually the culprit for much of our discomfort, as well as our growth.

The brain has a tremendous tendency to habituate, meaning to do the same thing over and over—which is great when you don't want to have to think about how you brush your teeth, but not so good when you need to think creatively about how to cope with a situation you've never been in before. That's why we so often tend to keep doing what we've already done, whether we get good results or not, and are slow to give up some destructive behaviors.

To add to the problem, part of habituation is the brain's tendency to look for patterns, to match current experience with the past. We think, *Oh, this is just like that thing that happened before.*

There's an adaptive reason for this habituation. The brain is always on and consumes a disproportionate part of the body's energy.

When the environment is stable, this autopilot serves us well. But during times of intense change, we have to fight against our brain's tendency to look at the situation and see the same old thing, when it's actually encountering something new.[1] This is especially true if the change involves something bad or painful.

As writer M.J. Ryan puts it, "The brain is hard-wired to scan for the bad, and when it inevitably finds negative things, they get stored immediately and are made available for rapid recall."[2] In contrast, positive experiences are usually registered through standard memory systems. They actually need to be held in conscious awareness for ten to twenty seconds for them to really sink in. In summary, your brain is like Teflon for positive experiences and Velcro for negative ones. This built-in bias puts a negative spin on the world and intensifies our stress and reactivity. Basically, the alarm section is constantly ready to react. And when it does, it's in the driver's seat, and you're going along for the ride. Like it or not, you're a passenger.

The Bilingual Brain

Your brain has two distinct parts, and the more you understand about it, the better you'll understand your past.

First of all, you and I have a bilingual brain. The left side of your brain speaks one language, and the right side speaks another. Sounds like the difference between a husband and wife and their style, doesn't it? Your right side is the emotional one. It controls intuitive, visual, and spatial reasoning. This side carries the music of experience. It stores the memory of the senses such as sounds, touch, and smell. It's full of pictures, like a silent movie. When you were being carried by your mother in her womb, the right side of your brain developed first. This side carries the nonverbal communication between mother and child. When you communicate using this side, you'll use facial expressions and body language, as well as singing and crying.

Your left side is the chatterbox. It does all the talking, and it remembers facts, statistics, and the vocabulary of events. It's full of words and narration. It's the seat of logic. But ask this side to describe or tell a story or tell an autobiographical narration, it needs to reach over to the right side and draw on the emotional memory that's stored there. That's what *should* happen. But here's the problem for those who have been traumatized: The left and right sides can't get together that well. The connection between the two sides has been hampered.[3]

The worst experience for a young child is neglect since it affects every part of the developing neurological system. When a child is born, he brings neurons in his brain that are just waiting to be stimulated and put into use. This promotes growth in the brain. Neglect affects every aspect of the developing neurological system. The lack of stimulation can cause atrophy to neurons that are ready at birth to go into service as the child experiences the new world. Chronic neglect will result in overall smaller brain size. Lack of stimulation also affects the size and strength of the neural networks within the brain.

And yes, it's true the brain of neglected children as well as those who were physically, emotionally, and sexually traumatized have been found to be smaller in overall size. Research indicates that chronic childhood abuse causes different and more intense changes in a person than an event which occurs in adulthood. It takes longer to overcome the impact of the abuse.[4]

Traumatized people have alterations in their brain. Traumatic events cause the left side (the cognitive or thinking side) and the right side (the emotional) to become disconnected from each other. Usually our body, emotions, and thoughts are all connected, but these events or traumas separate them. Left brain and right brain have to pull together, otherwise just one side is in charge. Both sides of the brain are meant to work together, but when one or the other shuts down, watch out! I work with many who have experienced some major upsetting events—these include accidents, shootings, and abuse. I know that each person's brain has been shaped by these experiences.

If you've ever experienced trauma, you know it's intrusive. Trauma interrupts and invades your life. It can also constrict and limit your life. Sometimes you alternate between the two—you find yourself caught between amnesia and reliving the trauma, between floods of intense, overwhelming feeling and arid states of no emotion whatsoever; between irritable, impulsive action and complete inhibition of action.[5] When you hear that someone has PTSD, this is what they are describing.

Let's repeat what can occur—indicate what you have experienced:

	Yes	No
Amnesia		
Reliving the experience		
Intense feelings		
No feelings		
Impulsive actions		
No action		

When something reminds a traumatized person of the past, their right brain reacts as if the traumatic event were happening in the present. Have you experienced this? The ability of this side of your brain is decreased; therefore, the brain is less able to do its left-brain functions. It can't distinguish a real threat from a false threat. It also limits people from putting into words what they feel. *They may think there is a danger when there isn't a danger* because the section of the brain that is supposed to analyze potential dangers isn't working. We experience triggers that take us back to the moment when the trauma happened.

I experienced a trigger for many years. I was a witness to a train wreck, and it happened right in front of me. The driver of a small car became impatient and drove between the arms that were down to prevent cars from going over the tracks. Before she could exit through the arms on the other side, the Amtrak train smashed into the side of the Volkswagen. I sat there watching and yelling for the train to stop—it didn't. Fortunately, the driver lived. I quickly drove to a phone (yes, this happened before cell phones) and reported what happened.

Unfortunately, I had to drive over the same tracks twice a day, five days a week. Each time I crossed over the tracks, I went into a hypervigilant mode. My car slowed down, almost to a complete stop. Did I plan to do this? No. Did I want to do this? No. My alarm section took over, and I became hyper-alert, which is a symptom of post-traumatic stress.

Because his or her left brain is not working very well, a person experiencing PTSD may not be aware that they are reexperiencing and reenacting the past—they are just furious, terrorized, engaged, ashamed, or frozen. The brain's left side can't get the words across to the right side to clarify what is occurring. And when words fail, haunting images capture the experience and return as nightmares and flashbacks in their brain's right side. Yes, your brain does all this. I've seen this in many places—most recently in those who experienced the shooting at the Route 91 concert in Las Vegas.

To sum up, those who experience post-traumatic stress have an overreactive alarm section in the right sides of their brains. They're activated to danger when there isn't any. It's like a car alarm system that keeps going off even when there's no danger, and the owner with the key isn't around to turn it off. With a brain scan, there is an abundance of lighting up on the right side and very little on the left, which implies that people are not necessarily thinking as much with the left side of their brain.[6] After the emotional storm passes, a person in this situation may look for somebody or something to blame for it.

Have you ever experienced a split brain? You may have vivid, graphic thoughts about what happened but have no emotion. Or you may experience intense emotions without the thoughts or actual memories. As one man said, "I feel like my brain has been disrupted, and one part transmits the AM and the other the FM. Sometimes there are holes in my memory like a slice was taken out. Other times I can't get those intrusive, unwanted memories to stop. I want them evicted! I can't remember what I want to remember, and I can't forget what I want erased." This struggle is shared by many.[7]

What happens when a threat is remembered? I've seen this first-hand with the victims of the Las Vegas shooting. I've seen their bodies tremble and their eyes glaze over. Their nervous system is overly activated by the past threat. Whatever event occurs, it seems to continue to float free in time rather than have roots and stability. This event comes uninvited into the present time and appears to the person as *This is happening now.* I've seen this in their facial expressions.

How can we switch to the CEO of our brain rather than allowing our alarm section to control us? There's good news—it's possible!

The Switch

First of all, your brain can grow no matter how old you are. It can grow new, positive pathways. It can help you see the upsets of life as challenges and thus calm down the alarm section of your brain. You don't need to be victimized by this section of your brain the rest of your life. Because of its location in the center of your brain, the alarm section reacts *fast*—even before the thinking part of your brain can kick in.[8] The portion of your brain that you want to access or be "in" is the CEO or the prefrontal cortex. This area allows you to solve complex problems, control your impulses, calm down intense emotions, shift your attention, and adapt to new, uncertain, or changing situations. It can also help you suppress automatic fearful or angry responses to stressful situations so that you can respond more effectively.[9] In order to activate the CEO in times of intense stress, consider the following steps:[10]

1. Acknowledge that you feel threatened or stressed.

2. Remind yourself that this is an automatic response and not necessarily a logical one.

3. Breathe slowly and evenly.

4. Become aware of triggers and warning signs.

5. After the situation occurs, replay it in your mind and re-create a rational and thoughtful outcome.[11]

Now, let's look at a few strategies more deeply.

Breathe deeply.

First, slow yourself down. Breathe in slowly, and hold your breath for four or five seconds. You can do this whether you're at home or at the mall. Do this several times, and you'll discover that you are more relaxed as well as thinking or moving at a different pace. When you hold your breath, your focus is no longer on the alarm or the pain or what has happened. Your breath is helping you relax, and your breath is helping you focus on the front part of your brain. Your entire body will begin to relax.

Dwell in truth.

Your mind actually adapts to whatever you dwell upon. Scripture instructs us, "Let the word of Christ dwell in you richly, teaching and admonishing one another in all wisdom, singing psalms and hymns and spiritual songs, with thankfulness in your hearts to God" (Colossians 3:16 ESV). So as you continue to breathe in and out, begin to repeat the following Scriptures. (Go ahead and read these aloud. Your brain needs to hear them as well as see them.)

> Be renewed in the spirit of your minds (Ephesians 4:23 ESV).

> Do not conform to the pattern of this world, but be transformed by the renewing of your mind. Then you will be able to test and approve what God's will is—his good, pleasing and perfect will (Romans 12:2).

> With minds that are alert and fully sober, set your hope on the grace to be brought to you when Jesus Christ is revealed at his coming (1 Peter 1:13).

Engage the present.

One of the best ways to move from one side of the brain to the other is to count backward from a hundred by sevens out loud. This is an exercise to help engage the hurting side of the brain and bring you back to the present.

Get it on paper.

Writing about painful experiences can be very helpful. Writing can help to boost your immune system and keep your body healthy. Writing, like any form of expression, can be a healing activity (remember the value of humor!). Writing about troubling experiences and the troubling aspects of your relationships helps you to see them more clearly and gives you a sense of mastery over your experiences. Once you put something down on paper, you may make connections you were not previously aware of and you may get in touch with feelings you haven't experienced before.[12]

Positive Deposits

Think of your mind or your brain as a bank. Like most banks, you can make deposits and withdrawals. Sometimes it's best to make a deposit, and there are times to make a withdrawal. My parents opened an account for me when I was two or three. I never made a deposit myself, but my parents took care of that for me. And because they made wise choices, the money they put in for me grew and grew over the years. What they did for me was for my benefit, and the results were positive. The amount deposited over the years grew. And at the proper time, we withdrew the money. There came a point in time when it was better to withdraw it than to leave it in.

We have all made deposits into our minds for years. Some of those deposits should never have been made. They were based upon distortion, misinformation, and even fear. When we discover we made a bad investment at a bank, the wise step is to immediately make a withdrawal. But too many hang on to what was deposited in their past, fail to check how it is doing, and end up losing money. The negative deposits may have been hurtful statements that were made to you or any form of abuse. The pain of those deposits grew and kept you living in your past. How you think and how you respond to others today is directly related to the thoughts which were deposited in your memory bank. Remember, *you can only draw on what was deposited.* It may be time to make some withdrawals so you can begin to live today.

I had no control over my deposits as a child. But as an adult, I do. So do you. It's time to clear out the account in your bank, and then make some new deposits. I want my brain to function in the way God intended. I think you do too.

Within the brain there are two related areas that are very important to the storage of memories. The *alarm section* is one, and the other portion is best described as your *brain's biographer* since it stores and retrieves conscious memories about what's going on now as well as events from the past and how you handled them and what happened. It's also called the hippocampus. Say that out loud—not hippopotamus, but hippocampus.

The alarm section has a specific job. It processes the intense and emotionally charged memories such as terror, and even the worst—horror. On the other hand, the biographer puts memories in the proper perspective. It gives the proper time sequence to events such as a beginning, middle, and end. But...when the alarm section is activated, the biographer's activity and functioning is diminished, and the past traumatic event continues to involve the present.[13] It's as though that portion of your brain takes over.

Uncharted Waters

We have a river not too far from where I live, and each year several people drown in it. They enter the water, but they don't know where the dangerous pools or submerged rocks are located. They're at risk since they don't know which section of the river is full of turbulence. They don't expect what they've run into.

I've waded a number of streams and rivers, especially in the Grand Teton National Park in Wyoming. Sometimes, I would be wading and a force of water would hit me, and I might fall over. The turbulence was there all along, but I just didn't see it.

Life is full of unchartered waters. Some people handle the waters well, and some do not. Those who are flexible expect to find those waters and are on the watch for them. Those people have the ability to adapt, survive, and eventually thrive. They are able to keep from getting stuck. They don't resist change but embrace it and use it. Resisting change, on the other hand, tears us down and has a negative effect on our thinking process.[14]

Whatever you're going through right now and whatever this change means to you, there's always a sense of loss of control. With change that comes from the outside, we aren't in charge of what's happening, and that's uncomfortable.[15] And what's worse is when this happens, it causes us to feel unsafe—especially if the change has been a traumatic one. Has this been your experience?

Messages from the environment go to both the alarm portion and other parts of your brain, but *they always get to the alarm part faster.* That's why we *must* be more skillful at learning to interpret the messages. The trick is to use the logical part of your brain to convince the scared part of yourself that there is no danger, at least none that you can't deal with.[16]

We need an emotional and cognitive helmet to protect our brain from disruption and concussion. Fortunately, we have that helmet. The prefrontal cortex, remember, helps us make decisions about right and wrong, or good and bad, and the consequences of our choices and actions. But here's the problem: It's not working as well as it should when you experience trauma or unexpected change. It's not running the show—the alarm section is in charge.

Managing Triggers

Most who have experienced trauma experience triggers or ambushes. As I worked with victims of the Las Vegas shooting, I kept hearing how triggers were a part of their life. One person I spoke with for several months after the tragedy told me that when the Fourth of July fireworks display began in the park near her house, her first inclination was to hide. The sound of the fireworks brought back unpleasant memories. The author of *Trust After Trauma* describes what you may be experiencing:

> Even simple matters, such as standing in line in a store or picking out a movie, can be problematic. Life is harder for you than for someone who hasn't been traumatized because of all the triggers in your environment and within yourself. You may feel sad and angry that you have to work harder than most people just to get through the day and you are entitled to both of these feelings.[17]

The author goes on to share a helpful exercise that you can try too:

Write the following:

1. Triggers you feel might be the easiest to endure.
2. Triggers you feel you might be able to handle after a few more months of healing.

3. Triggers you feel you might be able to confront in a few years (maybe).

4. Triggers you plan to avoid for the rest of your life.

Answer these questions and entitle a new page, "Trigger Chart" and draw lines to make four columns. Label them, from left to right, "Easiest to Handle," "Possibly Manageable Within a Year," "Possibly Manageable in the Distant Future" and "Impossible to Ever Handle."

Now take the answers from the questions above and place each trigger in the appropriate category. All of these steps will bring you into the front portion of your brain.

When you feel ready to confront a trigger, select one that you listed in column 1 of your Trigger Chart— a situation you judge one of the easiest to handle. Beginning with a more difficult trigger such as one in column 2 or 3, can be a setup for failure because no trigger situation, even one you classified as relatively easy to handle, is truly easy. You have to start somewhere, though, so it is best to start where you have the greatest chance of success.[18]

Once you have completed this process, write out what you think you can do to handle triggers. Find two safe people to share this with, and discuss two steps and write them out. One is how they can help you at this time, and secondly, how they can pray for you. Be honest about sharing your story and your feelings with them. Go back to the chart to help you move forward.

Trigger Chart

Easiest to Handle	Possibly Manageable Within a Year	Possibly Manageable in the Distant Future	Impossible to Ever Handle

One last thought about your body and especially your brain. Consider your spinal column. The spine is made up of 33 bones called vertebrae. These bones are stabilized by ligaments and separated by 23 intervertebral shock absorbers called disks. You have six disks in your neck, twelve in the middle of your back, and five in your lower back. This amazing design allows you to absorb the crushing blows your body experiences when running, jumping, or simply walking across a room. Without the shock absorbers, your back bones would slowly be crushed by pressure in the most common ritual of getting out of bed in the morning, let alone running a marathon or jumping in a gunny sack race on the Fourth of July. You were made to bounce. You were created with physical qualities that allow you to absorb the impact of shock and pressure without being crushed.

Your body also has the ability to heal itself. If you cut your hand, the wound will automatically begin to repair. This resilient healing process is constantly in motion in your body. It's what helps you rebound from wear and tear. Dying cells are replaced with new ones daily. Every 24 hours your body produces 200 billion new red blood cells. You feel refreshed after a good night's sleep, catch a second wind after a long day at work, and recover from a common cold or flu because your body is amazingly designed to bounce back.

We appreciate our bodies' resilience, especially when we suffer from an injury. But, for the most part, we are unaware of the awesome resilience movement going on under our skin. Have you ever wished your mind was created to be as resilient as your body? Wouldn't it be awesome if we could recover from life's crushing pressures and failures and bounce back the way our intervertebral disks do? When our life visions die, wouldn't it be comforting to know we can rejuvenate them the same way new red blood cells replace our dying ones?

The fact is you were made to bounce back not only physically, but also mentally, emotionally, and spiritually. And your brain was designed by a God of love, joy, and peace.[19]

Treat it well.

CHAPTER 12

Shaped by Your Thoughts

Our brain is a hormone factory. There are more than 100 of them (hormones, that is). The brain chemicals send messages to specific organs to complete specific tasks. Your brain (and everyone's) regulates, translates, and interprets those hormones. Remember these words: *regulate, translate,* and *interpret.* It's electrical code as hormonal output. When the output is high, you can tackle the world, but aging slows the process. The next statement is critical: As you get older, the production of hormones *slows down,* and if you don't have the right hormone level, your organs will slowly begin to stop functioning. This can lead to decline. And as the organs try to rectify the problem and create more of the good hormones, the stress hormone cortisol increases. All this affects the functioning of your organs, and it has a wearing effect on your brain. Your cognition, memory, and attention begin to wane.

If you're not as sharp as you used to be—I know I'm not!—the decline in your hormone levels is probably the reason for not being able to perform as well or why your brain fog seems to increase each year. That's the bad news part of this section. The good news is that it's possible to bring back proper levels of these hormones and actually resurrect old body parts—and this includes your brain. It will take work, patience, and probably a change in lifestyle. I have talked to a number of individuals who, for lack of a better phrase, have "given up." "What can I do about hormones at my age?" they wonder. Use them!

Were you aware that it's possible to rebuild former levels of hormones? It's true. You will need to work with your doctors to bring your body and your brain back to where your hormone levels were at their top level. Hormone supplements are effective as nutrients for a brain growing old. I've discussed this with a number of doctors who combine their medical practice with the use of supplements. The cost of these supplements is negligible when you discover the benefit. One of the key benefits is bringing your brain speed up to its former levels. Seek out experts in the field of supplements. It's worth the time and expense. There are some doctors who are focused upon the health and stimulation of your brain.

Brain Burn

There is one other factor that comes into play. Your illnesses. Your body's health influences the health of your brain. Every illness you experience has a detrimental effect upon your brain.

"Brain burn" occurs when you are sick. I've often wondered if I was impacted in this way since I was sick for almost a year when

I contracted polio. Illness impacts our brain. In fact, our body's health influences the health of our brain, and illness is not a friend to our brain. This is where brain burn comes in. If your brain is out of control, it could swell or dry out or be impacted by the environment. Blood diseases will impact your brain. The brain could be impacted negatively. And when this happens, our brain's abilities are compromised.

All this means you need to take a good look at your health and any illnesses you have or have had. How you take care of your physical health impacts the health of your brain. When was your last physical? Hopefully, it wasn't more than a year ago.

Get Moving!

Another way to stay healthy is exercise. But did you know exercise impacts the health of your brain in unexpected ways?

> The benefits of exercise include increased blood flow and new capillaries around neurons, increased production of new neurons and more interconnections between neurons, the protection of dopamine neurons from neurotoxins in the environment. Exercise also leads to elevations in nerve growth factors; elevations are there when you exercise. Exercise also affects prefrontal executive control processes; they're preferentially enhanced. It also brings about a positive balance in neurotransmitters just like antidepressants. In fact, a daily 1-mile walk reduces dementia risk by 50%.
>
> Important point: the brain's chemical messenger system is charged by exercise. The same neurotransmitters that are affected with antidepressants are also

affected by exercise. Psychiatrists now recommend combining meds and exercise.

Think of exercise on a continuum model. At one end, exercise is no longer necessary for survival; we don't have any lions we need to escape from, we don't have anything that makes us run on a regular basis to get away from something. On the other end of this continuum are the zealots; these people script their whole lives around compulsive exercising. And I use the word compulsive in a measured way because there's certain compulsivity about it and they want to have to exercise on a regular basis.[1]

How You Think = How You Feel

I've had a number of people tell me they allow their feelings to ruin their day. In one of the best books I've found on anxiety and worry, *Freeing Yourself from Anxiety*, the author discusses our struggles as well:

> Emotions arrive first and call the shots, causing you to react before you even know why. We fear feelings because often they make an experience worse before the rational mind catches up. You need to trust the notion that, although reason may come later to the party, it always shows up.[2]

When you find yourself upset emotionally, look for the link to your thoughts. It's like using the Internet. We have to click on the link to find what we're seeking. When you think about what you were thinking before you became upset, you'll probably find the link between your thoughts and emotions. When you click on a link that causes you to become upset, change the way you react to it. Rather than closing the link, browse awhile, navigate through your emotions, and welcome them.[3]

Now, this first step requires that you go beyond just identifying a thought. You need to begin with an emotion. Whenever you have an emotional reaction, label the emotion no matter what it is, whether it's negative or positive. Write it down.

Each emotion is actually a signal letting you know that something else is going on. Write *why* you are feeling the way you do. You could have more than one reason. Then ask yourself, "What are the thoughts that prompted this emotion?" It could have been a series of events or ideas. Try to put the thoughts you had in the sequence in which they occurred. Did your thoughts bother you, encourage you, or hinder your life in some way?

At the end of each day, review what you've written, and look for a pattern to your entries. Are there patterns to the thoughts or when they occurred? If you do this for a week, you may find a theme to your thoughts. Once you've identified the patterns, the next step is to evaluate them.

Are your thoughts accurate? It's important to be aware of what your thoughts are, what prompts them, and what their impact is on you and the people around you. Are your thoughts enhancing your life or detracting from it? Write your responses to these questions. Seeing the results will have a more powerful effect on you.

God knows our thoughts better than we do. Sometimes my thoughts puzzle me, confuse me, trouble me, surprise me, or delight me. But what is most important is what God thinks about my thoughts.

Negative thoughts develop negative emotional habits. It's a response you learn, and it becomes automatic because you use it so much. It's like an addiction, only a negative thinking pattern is the drug of choice.

Negative emotions, created by negative thoughts, are habits, just like your self-talk is a habit. They're not necessarily tied to your personality. It's not a matter of genes. And because of that, there's hope for change. What's been learned can be unlearned.

In *When Am I Going to Be Happy?* Penelope Russianoff points out:

> Emotional bad habits are losing games like playing against an opponent with loaded dice. As long as you keep playing with them, you will keep on losing.
>
> Strange—while negative emotions stick to us like tar, our positive, healthy, happy feelings are often fleeting and fragile. Good moods are shattered by the mildest reversals and instantly replaced by bad moods. A law of emotions seems to be at work here. Bad feelings drive out good feelings. The habit of looking at things negatively is so ingrained in some that they dismiss even happy experiences as no longer valid. They create "retroactive misery."[4]

We won't be able to really change our thoughts unless we understand how much our brain is involved. The changes we want to make involve changes in the brain. And this can happen.

Within the brain there is a section of memory banks (memory will be addressed elsewhere). When a thought is created within the brain or enters it, a section of the brain called the thalamus goes to work. The thalamus makes sense of the thought and runs it through the memory banks. There it's assessed by another portion of the brain, the amygdala. That's the storehouse of memories.

"When your thoughts are toxic or negative, you've handed off control to your emotions," which aren't always reliable. The amygdala has its place and its purpose, part of which is to alert us. "But unless it's steadied with nontoxic, balanced thoughts, the emotions it generates can dominate."[5]

Dorothy Finkelhor, in *How to Make Your Emotions Work for You*, says emotions are

> the motivating forces of our lives, driving us to go ahead, pushing us backward, stopping us completely, determining what we do, how we feel, what we want, and whether we get what we want. Our hates, loves, fears, and what to do about them are determined by our emotional structure. There is nothing in our lives that does not have the emotional factor as its mainspring. It gives us power, or makes us weak, operates for our benefit or to our benefit or to our detriment, for our happiness or confusion.[6]

Read and speak the following words out loud often. Let them remind you that God planned you and made you! See how that truth changes your emotions:

> You created my inmost being; you knit me together in my mother's womb. I praise you because I am fearfully and wonderfully made; your works are wonderful, I know that full well (Psalm 139:13-14).

> Before I formed you in the womb I knew you, before you were born I set you apart; I appointed you (Jeremiah 1:5).

> He chose us in [Christ] before the foundation of the

world, that we should be holy and blameless before him (Ephesians 1:4 ESV).

Thoughts—Good, Bad, or Otherwise

Thoughts—thousands of them a day created from the recesses of your brain. Many of which are healthy and good, while others are detrimental and limiting. Our thought life is a reflection of the depths of our brain. Some of our thoughts launch us into being healthy and productive, while others become intense and intrusive. Our lives either blossom or stagnate in response to our thoughts. Sometimes it seems like our brain is our friend, while other times it's our foe. Have you ever wondered what your brain is doing? Do your thoughts ever take over your will? Is your imagination working for you or against you?

God designed and gave us our minds—a unique blessing to the pinnacle of His creation. He also gave us instructions on how to protect and use that precious gift.

He says in His Word (emphasis added):

> Love the Lord your God with all your heart and with all your soul and with all your *mind* and with all your strength (Mark 12:30).

> Then he opened their *minds* so they could understand the Scriptures (Luke 24:45).

> Those who live according to the flesh have their *minds* set on what the flesh desires; but those who live in accordance with the Spirit have their *minds* set on what the Spirit desires (Romans 8:5).

> Do not conform to the pattern of this world, but be

transformed by the renewing of your *mind* (Romans 12:2).

Whatever is true, whatever is noble, whatever is right, whatever is pure, whatever is lovely, whatever is admirable—if anything is excellent or praiseworthy—*think* about such things (Philippians 4:8).[7]

Let's assume you have some negative thoughts flooding through your mind. Change each through a scriptural truth.

You're Enough

Over the past 40 years of counseling, I've very frequently heard one phrase: "I'm not enough." These words reflect the struggle many share. God wants us to experience the way in which He sees us. And yet, that experience seems to lie just out of our grasp. Imagine moving through each hour of the day with these thoughts and feelings hanging over you. Our brain was not created to create despair or depression. We are called to live a life of hope.

As negative thoughts begin to develop, they activate an emotional section of the brain. It's a negative—or toxic—thought, one of those insidious "downer" chemicals is released, stimulating the release of another, which stimulates the release of yet another.

Chemicals released by negative emotions can affect your brain's nerve cells, causing difficulty retrieving memories. That, in turn, suppresses the ability to remember and think in a constructive way. Chemicals released in the brain as a result of positive thoughts don't cause this kind of damage.

Toxic thoughts impact both emotional and physical balance. The hormones released can disrupt positive brain functioning, making it difficult for us to concentrate or focus.[8] Often these negative thoughts get stuck in our brain just like a broken record. You might be doing well in the present, but these past messages impact your brain.

The good news is that our thoughts can also create calm. When we're calm, we can control our emotions, reining them in before they spin out of control. Every positive or happy thought spurs your brain to action, releasing chemicals that make your body feel good.

Thoughts follow specific pathways in the brain. When a thought occurs, the thalamus goes to work making sense of the information and running it through the amygdala—which stores memories. Dr. Caroline Leaf notes:

> Remember that the amygdala (or the Smoke Alarm) is much like a library and is responsible for the first emotional response of any thought. It activates and arouses you to do something. If your "library" is filled with "books" that tell a story about not being able to cope with the incoming information, the response will be to react to the information based purely on an emotional level. This is why it is never wise to react to the first emotion you feel. It is a physiological response designed to alert and focus you, not to direct your actions.[9]

Guess what? When your thoughts are toxic or negative, you've handed off control to your emotions—chemical reactions that aren't always reliable. Part of the amygdala's purpose is to alert us. But unless it's steadied with nontoxic, balanced thoughts, the emotions it generates can dominate.[10] And that can cause a negative, even irrational response.

That's why memories, even those we don't consciously recall, can have powerful effects. Even if they're not readily accessed by the brain, so-called hidden memories still exist. Their information isn't lost; it's stored somewhere in the mind. It's as if those memories are burned onto the hard drive of the mind, and when we hit the right keys to trigger them, they reappear clearly to us.

Like so many other things, accessing memories is a biological process. We all have memories hidden somewhere beyond our conscious memory, blocked because the event was extremely painful or traumatic. It's as though God has built into the functioning of our mind the ability to repress emotionally painful material. Some of these memories stay there until our subconscious minds believe it's "safe" to access them. The majority of individuals have buried some of their experiences and have allowed the emotions of the past to dominate the present.

Which memories did you activate today? Were they negative or positive? Did they hinder your life or enhance it? This is why we want you to look at your past to make sure your past is not dominating the present. If so, you may discover that your brain is being dominated more by the past than by the present.

You can learn to control your thoughts that change your brain's chemistry, affect your emotions, and even influence your character. And that means you can have significant control over your physical well-being too. Pastor and author Charles Swindoll describes the power we have to direct our thoughts:

> Thoughts, positive or negative, grow stronger together when fertilized with constant repetition. That may explain why so many who are gloomy and gray stay in that mood, and why others who are cheery and enthusiastic continue to be so, even in the midst of difficult circumstances. Please do not misunderstand. Happiness (like winning) is a matter of right thinking,

not intelligence, age or position. Our performance is directly related to the thoughts we deposit in our memory bank. We can only draw on what we deposit.

What kind of performance would your car deliver if every morning before you left for work you scooped up handfuls of dirt and put it in your crankcase? The fine-tuned engine would soon be coughing and sputtering. Ultimately, it would refuse to start. The same is true of your life. Thoughts about yourself and attitudes toward others that are narrow, destructive and abrasive produce wear and tear on your mental motor. They send you off the road while others drive past.[11]

Science simply confirms what Scripture has been saying all along: We are shaped, in large part, by our thoughts. Why else would the great apostle Paul say, "Fix your thoughts on what is true and good and right" (Philippians 4:8 TLB)?

The Scriptures have much more to say about the act of thinking and our thought life. The words *think, thought,* and *mind* are used hundreds of times in the Bible. The writer of Proverbs 23:7 states succinctly, "As he thinks within himself, so he is" (NASB). Often the Scriptures refer to the heart as the source of our thoughts:

The heart of the righteous weighs its answers, but the mouth of the wicked gushes evil (Proverbs 15:28).

The things that come out of a person's mouth come from the heart, and these defile them. For out of the heart come evil thoughts—murder, adultery, sexual immorality, theft, false testimony, slander (Matthew 15:18-19).

> All the ways of a man are pure in his own eyes, but the
> Lord weighs the spirits (the thoughts and intents of
> the heart) (Proverbs 16:2 AMPC).

Our Creator designed us so that our thoughts have an impact on every aspect of life. Positive thoughts bring about positive effects. Negative thoughts take everything—from attitude to health—in the opposite direction. No wonder the author of Proverbs wrote, "A cheerful heart is good medicine, but a crushed spirit dries up the bones" (17:22).

Negative thoughts are a form of pollution to our body. What's more, our thoughts—good and bad—affect what we say and do. Jesus said,

> A good man brings good things out of the good stored
> up in his heart, and the evil man brings evil things out
> of the evil stored up in his heart. For the mouth speaks
> what the heart is full of (Luke 6:45).

Are your thoughts shaping you? Or are you shaping your thoughts? And what are your thoughts producing in your brain? Is your brain responding more to the past or the present?

If you're not in control of your mind, who is? Who has control of what you think—you or God?

CHAPTER 13

Rewriting the Past

Are you limited by your past? Have you ever felt as if life would be a lot easier if only those wounds and negative experiences from the past didn't keep interfering? Do you feel like you're *enough*? Maybe you don't like the identity you have, but you can't seem to rebuild.

I understand that. Sometimes hurts and issues from the past slow us down. You have to keep trying hard and expending so much effort before you finally start moving ahead. Excess emotional baggage can bog you down and rob you of blessing.

Some people are able to break free and move forward with their lives. Some cannot. Some struggle so hard just to make a slight bit of progress. Many are depressed because of what happened to them or because so many years were wasted before they finally came for counseling.

What Might Have Been

I've found that people deal with their emotional baggage in several inappropriate ways. Many of them are riddled with *regret over missed opportunities*. I often hear people say things like, "If only I had..." and "Oh, how I regret..." Another way we live our lives in the past is described by Dr. Jack Hayford as "the remembrance of reversals."[1] Reversals are similar to regrets, except the focus is on what might have been. "If only that hadn't happened," we might say, or "If only I could have done it differently." Sometimes to expediate the progress of growth and change, I ask counselees to make me a list of all their "if onlys" and regrets, so we can tackle each of them and eventually put them to rest.

If you're like me, you've revised some part of your past to an extent. We tend to rewrite it in one way or another, and sometimes what we remember isn't reliable or accurate. For those traumatized as children, painful experiences tattooed on their brain are accessed involuntarily. If that happened to you, it could be that the pain of your past is drawing you back. Rick Warren shared a helpful perspective for those with painful pasts: "We are products of our past, but we don't have to be prisoners of it. God's purpose is not limited by your past."[2]

Many people are driven by resentment and anger. They hold on to hurts and never get over them. Instead of releasing their pain through forgiveness, they rehearse it over and over in their minds. Many continue to stew in their pain, perpetuating the past.[3]

Painful experiences that weren't traumatic still can act as emotional magnets. For instance, if you have wounds from broken relationships with friends or family members, it could be you never received their acceptance or approval or forgiveness. We attempt to make others atone for what they did to us in the past. Blame and recrimination bring us to resentment, which leads to a lack of forgiveness, and we end up with a festering, painful memory. Issues like these can fasten their grip upon our mind and be like the bottom of an iceberg, deep and cold and foreboding.

Dan Allender wrote,

> Memory is to some degree a reconstruction of the past that is highly susceptible to erosion, bias and error. It is a mistake to consider one's memory completely accurate, no matter the level of emotional intensity or detail associated with the memories. We should maintain a tentative, open and non-dogmatic view toward all our memories.[4]

Memories start with an experience, but we often "update" them based on images formed or shaped by the intensity of our emotions. Details are altered, and some parts are reinforced and intensified, while others are diminished.

I've heard of family gatherings at which different members share their recollections of their past, while others look at one another and mutter, "That's not the way I remember it at all." Distortion can and does occur.

> When we begin to examine our recollections of our past closely, we find that they are malleable. That is not to say that the original memories are false; but what we thought were the "facts" of our past may turn out to be only a version of what happened to us, a "take" on our experiences...which we fixed in our minds long ago. As

long as these memories stay fixed, we are locked into an attitude, a general feeling, a guiding image of our past that makes it difficult to make changes. But when we recall and reexamine our memories, we realize just how constructed they are by our guiding image. So, they can be deconstructed, and when we do this, our feelings about the past can change also.[5]

We need to focus our brains on the positive past, not the negative. But many of the regrets I hear about are vain regrets. Whether we regret what was done to us by others or the sins we ourselves have committed, our looking back to the past only cripples the blessings of the present and detours us from entering the future. I'm not saying that we should never regret the past. There is a place and time for this—once! And then we must begin moving in a new direction.

A common response to the past is *renunciation.* We promise to change and do things differently. Past behaviors and attitudes are simply renounced, but they are not confronted and cleansed. My former pastor, Dr. Lloyd Ogilvie, put this so well when he wrote:

> We try to close the door on what has been, but all we do is suppress the dragons of memory. Every so often they rap persistently and want to come out into our consciousness for a dress rehearsal in preparation for a rerun in a new situation or circumstance. Renunciation of our memories sounds so very pious. The only thing wrong with it is that it doesn't work.[6]

We all have baggage and personal failures from the past. The past is past, and the events in that time frame can never be changed. But the effects can. You can get unstuck from the quicksand of past hurts by choosing to let God work in your life today.

Instead of dragging along the unnecessary baggage of regret, blame, and renunciation, have you ever tried rejoicing over the past? Rejoicing eventually brings release. Rejoicing over the past doesn't mean that you deny the hurtful incidents or the pain they brought you. Rather, you come to the place where you no longer ask *why*, but *how*: How can I learn from what happened to me and be a different person because of it?

Daring to Make a Change

Sometimes we are held back in our Christian life not only by a distorted image of God and of ourselves, but by experiences from the past. We exist, we can function, we understand our *eternal* destiny, but we're far from living a life of blessing in the here and now.

I remember a time when I was fishing the Snake River with a friend. We had been walking the river for about an hour when we found a place where two channels of the river converged—an ideal spot to fish. Since both my friend and I had waders on, we could walk through the water to any spot we chose. He chose to stand near the bank, and I headed out to a spot where the two channels came together.

As I stood there casting into the frothy water, I noticed that my feet were settling a bit deeper into the riverbed. But when I decided to move to another spot, I couldn't move my feet. I tried lifting one leg then the other, but both feet felt encased in cement, and nothing I tried seemed to work. I was stuck and stuck good.

The more I tried to extract my feet, the more I sank. Finally, in desperation, I hit upon the idea of lifting my feet out of the waders and then pulling the waders out of the mud. If I hadn't thought of taking my feet out of the boots first, I might still be stuck there!

Choosing to change is risky. The word *change* means to make different, to give a different course or direction, to replace one thing with another, to make a shift from one to another, to undergo transformation, transition, or substation. To many people, however, change is negative, something that implies inferiority, inadequacy, and failure. To them, the prospect of change might feel scary. No wonder so many people resist the idea of change. Who wants to feel inferior and inadequate?

Change is uncomfortable. We resist it even if it's for the better. It involves risk. It's risky to be a risk-taker. I know. I've taken a few risks. It's unsettling. It's unnerving. It produces some anxiety because we want to know the outcome of our choices in advance. There is a risk in seeking a new job. What if you're rejected, not just by one potential employer but by several? There is a risk in asking someone out on a date or asking someone to marry you. What if the person says no? That would hurt. But think of the blessing you could miss by not trying, by not asking, by not taking the risk.

I remember the risk of climbing out on a four-inch ledge to creep around a cliff jutting out over the icy water of a high-altitude lake. To add to the difficulty, I had to let go of one handhold to continue creeping along the ledge to reach the next handhold eight feet away. What if my foot slipped and I plunged 20 feet to the frigid water below? It was a risk. But I chose to take that risk to get to the inlet of the lake. It was worth it. Had I given up out of fear, I would have missed out on the joy of catching many brilliant, golden trout.

I also remember the risk of walking into a bank and asking for a loan of $2,000. It doesn't sound like much, but 44 years ago, when I was earning only $7,000 a year, $2,000 was a large amount to me. I intended to use the money to publish my own curriculum on marriage. I felt very strongly that this curriculum was needed so that others could teach marriage enrichment classes in their churches. But it still wasn't easy to take out that loan. Where was the assurance that others would buy these books? What if they didn't sell or other people didn't see the same benefit in them that I did?

But I took the risk. The plan was approved. The manuals were printed. They sold, and the monies funded the start-up of a nation-wide ministry of training and producing curriculum for churches. The risk was scary, but the blessings enjoyed by thousands of couples over the years have been well worth it.

The Story of You

You and I have stories to tell. Some good and some not so good. Some are full of memories. One of the best descriptions I have heard of the importance of telling our stories is found in the book *Bounce,* by Aaron Fruh:

> If I have buried the truth of my story, I become but a shell of a person living in denial of the human experience with all of its pain and pleasure. For many, painful memories are like unseen tent pegs driven deep into their souls, tethering the bonds of their reluctant encampments. They long to move on as sojourners, but because of an unwillingness to understand their stories, they eventually become settlers, surrounded by so much mental baggage they can't go anywhere.

> If you've become a settler in suffering, it's time to become a sojourner, pull up the tent pegs, and move on. Liquidating some mental real estate is the first step in your resilience plan. You need to find the meaning for what has happened to you, and in finding that meaning you'll find healing. A good place to start is writing your story. This statement, which has been

attributed to several authors, rings true to me: "We don't write to be understood; we write to understand."[7]

In what way might you be a shell? Watch out for mental baggage that ties you to your past. It's important that you let go of your past identity (based on inaccurate messages about yourself) and that you build a new identity based on the unconditional love and acceptance of God. To do so, you need unconditional love and your true, God-given identity. Once you decide which identity is of greater value, you need to let go of one and grab for the other. His voice is better than the other voices.

Dr. Paul Tournier compares Christian growth to the experience of swinging from a trapeze. The man on the trapeze clings to the bar because it is his security. When another trapeze bar swings into view, he needs to release his grip on one bar in order to leap to the other. It's a scary process. Similarly, God is swinging a new trapeze bar into your view. It is a positive, accurate, new identity based on God's Word. But in order to grasp the new, you have got to release the old. You may have difficulty relinquishing the familiarity and security of your old identity. But think of what you will gain.[8]

You and I are like a bank account that has insufficient funds. We're always in debt. And we end up in despair. But if we're walking with Christ, we have been saved by grace and are made alive by grace. In his book *Love Beyond Reason*, John Ortberg gives a clear description of what God's grace has done:

> This is grace for anyone who's ever despaired over sin. This is the removal of our mountain of moral indebtedness. If you've ever felt that gap between reality and who you're called to be, ever felt like you can't close it...this is grace for you. God took our indebtedness and guilt and nailed it to the cross. He erased

the bill, destroyed the IOU, so you are free. Unburdened. Cleansed. You can live with a heart as light as a feather. Today—no matter what you did yesterday. This is the wonder of grace.[9]

Grace is totally free. It cannot be bought. It is undeserved, unearned, and cannot be repaid. In Ephesians 2:4-5, the apostle Paul tells us, "Because of his great love for us, God, who is rich in mercy, made us alive with Christ even when we were dead in transgressions—it is by grace you have been saved."

God doesn't say...

"I love you because..."

"I love you since..."

"I will love you if..."

"I will love you when..."

"I will love you provided..."

In no way is God's love conditional.[10] The voices in our mind are not true.

Simply put, grace extends favor and kindness to one who doesn't deserve it and can never earn it. Every time you think of the word *grace*, think *undeserved, undeserved, undeserved.*

The greatest gift of His grace was given to us through Christ.

Because of Christ's redemption,

I am a new creation of infinite worth.

I am deeply loved,

I am completely forgiven,

I am totally pleasing,

I am totally accepted by God,

I am absolutely complete in Christ.

When my performance

Reflects my identity in Christ,

That reflection is dynamically unique.
There has never been another person like me
In the history of mankind,
Nor will there ever be.
God has made me an original,
One of a kind,
A special person.[11]

Read these statements out loud each day for a week and discover the difference these true statements will make in your life and how you will see yourself. You will indeed have a new identity. The grooves that these words cut into your brain can be a blessing in your life.

Here is a prayer that may assist you:

> *Lord, I am at the place of asking You to take over my thought life, my inner dialogues, and my imagination, and not only clean them up, but give me the power to control my thoughts. I am learning which thoughts cause me the most grief and which ones help me. I have to admit to You that I am a creature of habit, and I know I have spent years developing this type of negative thinking. I want to communicate better with others and with myself, and I need Your help. I ask You to cause me to be very aware of what I am thinking from time to time. Help me not to fall back into being negative about myself because of this lapse. Help me to be patient with myself and with You. Thank You for hearing me and accepting me; and thank You for what You will do for my thought life and inner dialogues in the future.*

Pray this prayer out loud each day for a month and notice the difference. And remember, as the apostle Paul reminds us, "God's grace is sufficient for me and His strength is made perfect in my weakness; therefore, I will glory in my weakness that the power of Christ may rest upon me" (2 Corinthians 12:9).

What a difference these words can make in your life.

The Fantasy of a Changed Life

Thomas Edison did not just sit down and invent the lightbulb. He first lay on the couch in his workshop and filled his mind with fantasies. Debussy created some of his music by imaging reflections of the sun on a river.

Fantasy can be a form of escape, rescuing us from the daily doldrums and leading us away from responsibilities, pain, and disillusionment. But fantasy, as Edison and Debussy showed, can also lead us to invent a machine! Fantasies can be powerful magnets drawing out our abilities and strengths to unlock problems and tear down barriers blocking our progress.

Fantasy can also be used to help heal your detrimental memories and free you from self-condemnation. If you want a future that's different from your past, you have to start by envisioning change. Imagine what it would look like to be free!

Maybe you've been believing lies about yourself: *I can't do that. It's over my head. If I try that, I'm going to fail.* That feeling of inferiority limits your efforts and keeps you caged and shackled. But you don't have to stay in chains. Imaging and prayer, followed with action, are the keys. Picture yourself facing some overwhelming situation, with Jesus standing beside you. He takes the first step forward. See yourself taking one step to bring yourself up beside Jesus. He takes another step, and you again move up beside Him. Saturating your mind—imaging the presence of God—can free you from the fear of failure. It takes time, work, and effort. Scripture tells us to expect this: "With minds that are alert and fully sober," says 1 Peter 1:13, "set your hope on the grace to be brought to you when Jesus Christ is revealed."

Today, I challenge you to give that kind of positive fantasy a try! Find a quiet spot where you can sit without fear of interruption. Sit comfortably, with your feet on the floor.

Focus on the rhythm of your breathing. Concentrate on this.

Relax and recognize that you are in a quiet place. Visualize any tension you feel as knots or tourniquets. See them coming undone.

Our minds can create images so realistic they chart the direction we choose to move, for our actions and feelings begin there. These fantasies, or images, can be used to bring about the positive changes we seek in our lives.

The finest description of imaging I have read is the following:

> Imaging, the forming of mental pictures or images, is based on the principle that there is a deep tendency in human nature to ultimately become precisely like that which we imagine or image ourselves as being. An image formed and held tenaciously in the conscious mind will pass presently, by a process of mental osmosis, into the unconscious mind. And when it is accepted firmly in the unconscious, the individual will strongly tend to have it, for then it has you. So powerful is the imaging effect on thought and performance that a long-held visualization of an object or goal can become determinative.[12]

Imaging is positive thinking carried one step further. In imaging someone does not merely think about a hoped-for goal; they "see" or visualize it with tremendous intensity, reinforced by prayer. Imaging is a kind of laser beam of the imagination, a shaft of mental energy in which the desired goal or outcome is pictured so vividly by the conscious mind that the unconscious mind accepts it and is activated by it. This releases powerful internal forces that can bring about astonishing changes in the life of the person who is doing the imaging.[13]

High blood pressure patients also make use of this technique. They practice relaxation exercises as well as imagery. In their imagery, they see their blood vessels as pipes. They visualize their muscles tightening and making the pipes narrower, so the blood has more difficulty getting through. Then they see their medication releasing the muscles, so the heart has an easier time in its work of pumping the blood through these vessels. Guided imagery has proven to be a safe and effective way of raising an individual's tolerance to pain as well as freeing up the nervous system to maximize the healing processes of the body.

I have talked to many who have confessed their sins to God, asked Him to forgive them, and in some cases even made restitution. They realize intellectually that God has forgiven them, but emotionally they do not feel forgiven. They still feel unworthy and guilty. I usually suggest that they do the following imagery exercise to help them find the freedom from guilt they seek:

> Sit back in your chair and close your eyes. Visualize a large blackboard with a mass of meaningless words and phrases written on it. As you look more closely, this mass of words begins to spell out the acts or behaviors for which you do not feel forgiven. They now stand out clearly and boldly among the other words and phrases.
>
> Now, visualize Jesus Christ standing at the board. He is sweeping a damp sponge across that blackboard, wiping it clean. He keeps on until it is so clean that

something fresh and new and meaningful can be written on it. God is erasing your past sin and failures so you can start again.

Now, visualize Jesus beckoning you to come to the blackboard. He asks you to place your hand in His, and He says, "I want you to see that the board has really been wiped clean. Feel My hand cleaning the board, and believe that it is becoming clean and new again." You feel His hand cleaning the board, and now it begins to dawn on you: Jesus is actually doing this for you.

Then, visualize Jesus turning to you, placing His hand on your shoulder, and saying, "You are forgiven. Experience My forgiveness as a part of your life. Live your life as a forgiven person." By this action, He is also telling you to forgive yourself, for there is no need to keep count of the errors on the blackboard. They no longer exist. It is as though someone hit the Erase button on the calculator.

You need to run this picture and sequence through your mind again and again until, through prayer, you experience the acceptance and forgiveness that are yours.

CHAPTER 14

Let the Spirit Lead You

People sometimes ask, "Is it possible to get a brain or mind transplant?" We all laugh...at first. But the idea isn't without appeal. It sometimes seems it would be easier to start over with a clean slate, rather than continue enduring the turmoil that occurs inside our minds or go through all the work it takes to change these entrenched patterns from the past. According to Scripture, it is possible to have a change in our mind.

The Bible records that "the LORD saw how great the wickedness of the human race had become on the earth, and that *every inclination of the thoughts of the human heart* was only evil all the time" (Genesis 6:5, emphasis added). Isn't it interesting that the first place human beings turned away from God was in their thoughts?

Centuries later, the apostle Paul was still stating the same problems. "Although they knew God, they neither glorified him as God nor gave thanks to him, but *their thinking became futile and their foolish hearts were darkened*" (Romans 1:21, emphasis added). Wrong thinking can develop from what affected us in our past.

The solution isn't to try to control the content of your mind on your own. Instead, choose to give God the control. Romans 8:5-7 warns:

> Those who live according to the flesh have their minds set on what the flesh desires; but those who live in accordance with the Spirit have their minds set on what the Spirit desires. The mind governed by the flesh is death, but the mind governed by the Spirit is life and peace. The mind governed by the flesh is hostile to God; it does not submit to God's law, nor can it do so.

Our goal should be to let our mind be controlled by the Spirit. We should want to set it on what God wants. Just as a reminder, the fruit of the Spirit is "love, joy, peace, patience, kindness, goodness, faithfulness, gentleness, self-control" (Galatians 5:22-23 ESV). So much of what occurs in our life is because of the fruit of the Spirit.

Here's the good news. *What we think can be reversed.* Like a boat that's been moving in the wrong direction, you can turn your thinking around and start moving your life in another direction. You will appreciate this. Others will appreciate this. Your brain will appreciate this as well.

Have you struggled to change your thought life? Of course, you have. We all have. Maybe you've tried different approaches or programs, prayed about it, been prayed over, and so on. But you still struggle. So do I. Any change you want to make is not a simple step-by-step process or an overnight event. That's because your brain wasn't designed to make permanent changes suddenly.

The brain, all three pounds of it, follows patterns of habits established over the years. Can you imagine this small portion of your body controlling you? We can't expect this unique organ of the body—with its billions of neurons and millions of pathways, circuits, and memory cells—to erase what it's built over the years, replacing it with entirely new thinking and new wiring instantaneously. When we try to make sudden changes, we ask the brain to do something it wasn't designed to do. So when we begin changing old patterns, we should expect old ways of thinking and talking to challenge the new. We're likely to tell ourselves things like, "This won't work."

But this is good. It shows the new approach is working. You've disrupted that old way of thinking, and now it's resisting the change. God's Word has much to say about your brain:

> Do not be conformed to this world (this age), [fashioned after and adapted to its external, superficial customs], but be transformed (changed) by the [entire] renewal of your mind [by its new ideals and new attitude], so that you may prove [for yourselves] what is the good and acceptable and perfect will of God, even the thing which is good and acceptable and perfect [in His sight for you] (Romans 12:2 AMPC).

Read this Scripture verse aloud several times. Your brain needs to not only *see* the words but *hear* them as well. You've heard this suggestion before, and it does make a difference.

The renewal here is the spirit of the mind. Under the controlling power of the Holy Spirit, a believer can direct his thoughts and energies toward God. The renewing of the mind is the adjustments of the person's thinking and outlook on life so that these conform to the mind of God.

We want our mind to be focused on Christlike thoughts, as we're instructed in Colossians 3:1-2: "If then you have been raised with Christ, seek the things that are above, where Christ is, seated at the right hand of God. *Set your minds on things* that are above, not on things that are on earth" (ESV, emphasis added). The phrase "set your minds on" means to think on or focus on.

Your brain's ability to change was greatest in childhood and adolescence. Don't be discouraged if you're a few decades beyond that time period! Change as an adult is still very possible—even now. One of my favorite authors, John Ortberg, is a pastor who is very insightful and practical. In his book *The Me I Want to Be*, he writes this:

> Even twenty years ago, researchers thought the adult brain was genetically determined and structurally unchangeable. But they have since found that even into adulthood the brain is amazingly changeable— it has neuroplasticity. Which synapses remain and which ones wither away depends on your mental habits. Those that carry no traffic go out of business like bus routes with no customers. Those that get heavily trafficked get stronger and thicker. The mind shapes the brain. Neurons that wire together fire together. In other words, when you practice hope, love or joy, your mind is actually, literally, rewiring your brain![1]

In order for thinking to change, we need a new vision. You may call it a goal. It involves identifying the way you want your thinking to be. It involves creating a new pattern of thinking and new phrases. But it's more than that.

In *Living Above the Level of Mediocrity*, Chuck Swindoll describes what developing a vision really entails:

> Vision is the ability to see God's presence, to perceive God's power, to focus on God's plan, in spite of the obstacles...Vision is the ability to see above and beyond the majority. Vision is perception—reading the presence and power of God's into one's circumstances. I sometimes think of vision as looking at life through the lens of God's eyes, seeing situations as He sees them. Too often we see things not as they are, but as we are. Think about that. Vision has to do with looking at life with a divine perspective, reading the scene with God in clear focus. Whoever wants to live differently in "the system" must correct his or her vision.[2]

Scripture tells us that our minds need to be changed before we can see with God's eyes: "Do not be conformed to this world...but be transformed (changed) by the [entire] renewal of your mind [by its new ideals and its new attitude], so that you may prove [for yourselves] what is the good and acceptable and perfect will of God, even the thing which is good and acceptable and perfect" (Romans 12:2 AMPC).

And the more you learn, the more you'll grow and change.

You don't have to take these steps by yourself. Let God change you from the inside out. And let the Holy Spirit guide your brain.

After all is said and done in this book, it comes down to this: Our calling as believers is to allow Jesus to be at the center of our life. No matter who we are or where we are, our calling is to reflect the fruit of the Spirit in our life and...in everything we do!

Notes

Chapter 1—How's Your Brain?

1. Kayt Sukel, ed., *The Brain: The Ultimate Guide* (New York: Ben Harris, 2015), 7, 27.

2. Dr. Caroline Leaf, *Switch on Your Brain: The Key to Peak Happiness, Thinking, and Health* (Grand Rapids, MI: Baker Publishing, 2015), 16, 99.

3. Aaron Fruh, *Bounce: Learning to Thrive Through Loss, Tragedy and Heartache* (Grand Rapids, MI: Baker Books, 2017), 22-23.

4. David Eagleman, *The Brain: The Story of You* (New York: Pantheon Books, 2015).

Chapter 2—Getting to Know Your Brain

1. John B. Arden, *Rewire Your Brain: Think Your Way to a Better Life* (Hoboken, NJ: Wiley Publishing, 2010), adapted, 43-44.

2. Daniel Amen, *Memory Rescue: Supercharge Your Brain, Reverse Memory Loss, and Remember What Matters Most* (Wheaton, IL: Tyndale Momentum, 2017), 13-16.

3. Tamar E. Chansky, *Freeing Yourself from Anxiety: 4 Simple Steps to Overcome Worry and Create the Life You Want* (Boston, MA: Da Capo Press, 2012), 4.

4. Sherri Keffer, *Intimate Deception: Healing the Wounds of Sexual Betrayal* (Grand Rapids, MI: Revell, 2018), 170-71.

5. Bessel van der Kolk, *The Body Keeps the Score: Brain, Mind, and Body in the Healing of Trauma* (New York: Viking, 2014), 61-64.

6. Chansky, *Freeing Yourself from Anxiety,* 5.

7. Ibid., 4.

8. Michael J. Scott, *Moving on After Trauma: A Guide for Survivors, Family, and Friends* (New York: Routledge, 2008), 23-25.

9. Judith Herman, *Trauma and Recovery: The Aftermath of Violence—from Domestic Abuse to Political Terror* (New York: Basic Books, 1982), 47.

10. Chansky, *Freeing Yourself from Anxiety,* 5.

11. Ibid.

12. Laurence Gonzales, *Surviving Survival: The Art and Science of Resilience* (New York: W.W. Norton & Co., 2012), 25-27.

13. van der Kolk, *The Body Keeps Score*, 80.

14. Jeffrey M. Schwartz, *Brain Lock: Free Yourself from Your Obsessive-Compulsive Behavior* (New York: Harper Perennial, 2016), 52.

Chapter 3—Hardwired to Change

1. "Hardwire," www.lexico.com/en/definition/hardwire.

2. John B. Arden, *Rewire Your Brain: Think Your Way to a Better Life* (Hoboken, NJ: Wiley Publishing, 2010), 8-9.

3. Ibid., 10.

4. Aaron Fruh, *Bounce: Learning to Thrive Through Loss, Tragedy and Heartache* (Grand Rapids, MI: Baker Books, 2017), 21-23.

5. Caroline Leaf, *Who Switched Off My Brain?* (Nashville: Thomas Nelson, 2009), 16, 99.

6. Zaldy S. Tan, *Age-Proof Your Mind: Detect, Delay, and Prevent Memory Loss—Before It's Too Late* (New York: Grand Central Life & Style, 2006), 6.

7. *Combating Memory Loss: Common Problems and Treatments*, A Special Report by the editors of *Mind, Mood & Memory* in cooperation with Massachusetts General Hospital (2020).

8. Gail Sheehy, *New Passages: Mapping Your Life Through Time* (New York: Ballantine Books, 1996), 424-26.

9. Nursing Assistant Central, "100 Fascinating Facts You Never Knew About the Human Brain," www.scribd.com/document/82778570/100-Fascinating-Facts-You-Never-Knew-About-the-Human-Brain-Nursing-Assistant-Central.

10. Time Special, "Forgetting Childhood," *The Science of Memory: The Story of Our Lives*, December 21, 2018, 38.

Chapter 4—The Basics of Brain Refreshment

1. K.C. Wright, "Mediterranean Diet Improves Cognition, Memory and Brain Volume," *Today's Dietician* 20, no. 6 (June 2018): 40, www.todaysdietitian.com/newarchives/0618p40.shtml.

2. Kim E. Innes, "Meditation and Music Improve Memory and Cognitive Function in Adults with Subjective Cognitive Decline: A Pilot Randomized Controlled Trial," *Journal of Alzheimer's Disease* 56, no. 3 (January 2017): 899-916, doi: 10/3233/JAD-160867.

3. H.J. Trappe and G. Voit, "The Cardiovascular Effect of Musical Genres: A Randomized Controlled Study on the Effect of Compositions by W.A. Mozart, J. Strauss, and ABBA" *Deutsches Arzerblatt International* 113, no. 20 (May 20, 2016): 347-52. doi: 10.3238/arztebl 2016.0347.

4. H.P. Lee, Y.C. Liu, and M.F. Lin, "Effects of Musical Genres on the Psycho-Physiological Responses of Undergraduates," *Hu Li Za Zhi: The Journal of Nursing* 63, no 6 (December 2016): 77-88, doi: 10.6224/JN 63.6.77.

5. M. Herdener, et al, "Musical Training Induces Functional Plasticity in Human Hippocampus," *Journal of Neuroscience* 30, no. 4 (January 27, 2010): 1377-84, doi: 10.1523/JNEURO.

6. S. Sheldon and J. Donahue, "More Than a Feeling: Emotional Cues Impact the Access and Experience of Autobiographical Memories," *Memory and Cognition* 45 (February 27, 2017): 731-44, doi: 10.3758/s13421-017-0691-6.

7. Gini Graham Scott, *30 Days to a More Powerful Memory* (New York: Amacom, 2007), 20-22.

8. Ibid., 50.

9. Ibid., 51.

10. George W. Rebok, "Ten-Year Effects of the Advanced Cognitive Training for Independent and Vital Elderly Cognitive Training Trial on Cognition and Every-day Functioning in Older Adults," *Journal of the American Geriatrics Society* 62, no 1. (2014): 16-24, doi: 10.1111/jgs. 12607.

11. Daniel Amen, *Memory Rescue: Supercharge Your Brain, Reverse Memory Loss, and Remember What Matters Most* (Wheaton, IL: Tyndale Momentum, 2017), 294-95.

12. Gini Graham Scott, *30 Days to a More Powerful Memory* (New York: Amacom, 2007), 63.

13. Bronwyn Fox, *Power Over Panic* (Upper Saddle River, NJ: Prentice Hall, 2001), 116-17.

14. John B. Arden, *Rewire Your Brain: Think Your Way to a Better Life* (Hoboken, NJ: Wiley Publishing, 2010), 77.

Chapter 5—Right and Left

1. Bill and Pam Farrel, *Men are Like Waffles, Women are Like Spaghetti: Understanding and Delighting in Your Differences* (Eugene, OR: Harvest House Publishers, 2015), 11.

2. Bessel van der Kolk, *The Body Keeps the Score: Brain, Mind, and Body in the Healing of Trauma* (New York: Viking, 2014), 44-45.

3. Sharon Begley, *Train Your Mind, Change Your Brain* (New York: Ballantine, 2007), 8.

Chapter 6—Who You Are Inside

1. Elena Welsh, Ph.D., *Trauma Survivors Strategies for Healing* (Alethea Press, 2018), 103.

2. Marty Olsen Laney, *The Introvert Advantage: How Quiet People Can Thrive in an Extrovert World* (New York: Workman Publishing Company, 2002), 70-71.

3. Ibid., 86.

4. Ibid., 85-86.

5. Ibid., 49.

Chapter 7—Thanks for the Memories...I Think

1. *Combating Memory Loss Common Problems and Treatments*, 2018 Report, 85. A Special Report published by the editors of *Mind, Mood & Memory* in cooperation with Massachusetts General Hospital.

2. Ibid.

3. Ibid., 81.

4. Marc Pleugar, *The Perfect Brain Book* (Reader's Digest), adapted, 122-25.

5. Kasee Bailey, "5 Powerful Health Benefits of Journaling," July, 31, 2018. https://intermountainhealthcare.org/blogs/topics/live-well/2018/07/5-powerful-health-benefits-of-journaling.

6. Tanya Lewis, "Bilingual People are like Brain Bodybuilders," *Live Science*, November 12, 2014. http://www.livescience.com/48721-bilingual-brain-bodybuilders.html.

7. Mia Nacamulli, "The Benefits of the Bilingual Brain," *TED Ed*, June 2, 2015, https://ed.ted.com/lesson/how-speaking-multiple-languages-benefits-the-brain-mia-nacamulli.

8. Bonnie Sparrman, *60 Ways to Keep Your Brain Sharp* (Eugene, OR: Harvest House Publishers, 2018), 125.

9. Ibid., 163.

10. Elena Welsh, Ph.D., *Trauma Survivors Strategies for Healing* (Alethea Press, 2018), 55.

Chapter 8—Rehearse, Repeat

1. Gini Graham Scott, *30 Days to a More Powerful Memory* (New York: Amacom, 2007), 145.

2. Geoff Colvin, *Talent Is Overrated* (New York: Portfolio Hardcover, 2008).

3. Ibid., 67-68.

4. H. Norman Wright, *A Better Way to Think* (Grand Rapids, MI: Revell, 2011), 118-23.

5. Zaldy S. Tan, *Age-Proof Your Mind: Detect, Delay, and Prevent Memory Loss—Before It's Too Late* (New York: Grand Central Life & Style, 2006), 200-15.

6. Ibid., 218.

7. Ibid., 218-19.

8. Megan Devine, *It's OK That You're Not OK: Meeting Grief and Loss in a Culture That Doesn't Understand* (Boulder, CO: Sounds True, 2017), 136.

Chapter 9—Worry on the Mind

1. Edward M. Hallowell, *Worry: Hope and Help for a Common Condition* (New York: Ballantine Books, 1977), 73-74.

2. Ibid., 5.

3. Jeffrey M. Schwartz, *Brain Lock: Free Yourself from Your Obsessive-Compulsive Behavior* (New York: Harper Perennial, 2016), xxii.

4. Ibid.

5. Ibid., 25.

6. H. Norman Wright, *Overcoming Worry & Fear* (Torrance, CA: Aspire Press, 2014), 103-08.

7. Max Lucado, *Come Thirsty* (Nashville, TN: Thomas Nelson, 2010), 106.

8. Ibid., 157.

9. Ibid., 6.

10. Business 901, June 23, 2015, "Overcoming OCD in Sales Efforts," https://business901.com/blog1/overcoming-ocd-in-sales-efforts.

11. Hallowell, *Worry,* adapted, 67.

12. Ibid., 23.

Chapter 10—The Grieving Brain

1. Joanne T. Jozefowski, *The Phoenix Phenomenon* (Northvale, NJ: Jason Aronson, Inc., 2001), 17.

2. "Greenlight," *The Rookie* (Los Angeles, CA: ABC), March 16, 2019.

3. Carol Staudacher, *Beyond Grief* (Oakland, CA: New Harbinger, 1987), 47.

4. Megan Devine, *It's OK That You're Not OK: Meeting Grief and Loss in a Culture That Doesn't Understand* (Boulder, CO: Sounds True, 2017), 129.

5. Ibid., 126.

6. Terry L. Martin and Kenneth J. Doka, *Men Don't Cry…Women Do: Transcending Gender Stereotypes of Grief* (Philadelphia, PA: Bruner/Mazell, 2000), 35.

7. Ibid., 63-64.

8. Lewis B. Smedes, *Forgive and Forget* (New York: Harper & Row, 1984), 37.

Chapter 11—When It Hurts Too Much

1. Bessel van der Kolk, *The Body Keeps Score: Brain, Mind and Body in the Healing of Trauma* (New York: Penguin Books, 2015), 52.

2. M.J. Ryan, *How to Survive Change You Didn't Ask For* (Newburyport, MA: Conari Press, 2014), 20.

3. Heather Davediuk Gingrich, Ph.D., *Restoring the Shattered Self: A Christian Counselor's Guide to Complex Trauma* (Downers Grove, IL: IVP Academic, 2013), 38-39.

4. van der Kolk, *The Body Keeps Score*, 255.

5. Ibid., 52.

6. Judith Herman, *Trauma and Recovery: The Aftermath of Violence—from Domestic Abuse to Political Terror* (New York: Basic Books, 1982), 42-43.

7. Melanie Greenberg, *The Stress-Proof Brain: Master Your Emotional Responses to Stress Using Mindfulness and Neuroplasticity* (Oakland, CA: New Harbinger, 2017), 60-61, 3.

8. Ibid., 65.

9. Ibid., 17.

10. Ryan, *How to Survive Change You Didn't Ask For*, 22-23.

11. Nancy Moyer, MD, "Amygdala Hijack: When Emotion Takes Over," *Healthline,* April 22, 2019, adapted, https://www.healthline.com/health/stress/amygdala-hijack#overview.

12. Aphrodite T. Matsakis, *Trust After Trauma: A Guide to Relationships for Survivors and Those Who Love Them* (Oakland, CA: New Harbinger Publications, 1998), 9-10.

13. Babette Rothschild, *The Body Remembers* (New York: W.W. Norton, 2000), 12.

14. M.J. Ryan, *How to Survive Change You Didn't Ask For: Bounce Back, Find Calm in Chaos, and Reinvent Yourself* (Newburyport, MA: Conari Press, 2014), 4-5, 10.

15. Ibid., 28-29.

16. Ibid., 57.

17. Matsakis, *Trust After Trauma*, 105.

18. Ibid., 122.

19. Aaron Fruh, *Bounce: Learning to Thrive Through Loss, Tragedy and Heartache* (Grand Rapids, MI: Baker Books, 2017), 20-21.

Chapter 12—Shaped by Your Thoughts

1. Richard Restak, *Optimizing Brain Fitness* (Chantilly, VA: The Great Courses, 2011), 42-43.

2. Tamar E. Chansky, *Freeing Yourself from Anxiety: 4 Simple Steps to Overcome Worry and Create the Life You Want* (Boston, MA: Da Capo Press, 2012), 159.

3. Ibid.

4. Penelope Russianoff, *When Am I Going to Be Happy? How to Break the Emotional Bad Habits that Make You Miserable* (New York: Bantam, 1988), 7.

5. Ibid., 50-52.

6. Dorothy Finkelhor, *How to Make Your Emotions Work for You* (New York: Berkley, Medallion Books, 1973), 23-24.

7. Stan Toler, *ReThink Your Life* (Indianapolis: Wesleyan Publishing House, 2000), 30-31.

8. Don Colbert, *Deadly Emotions* (Nashville: Thomas Nelson, 2003), 24-27.

9. Dr. Caroline Leaf, *Switch on Your Brain: The Key to Peak Happiness, Thinking, and Health* (Grand Rapids, MI: Baker Publishing, 2015), 9-10.

10. Ibid., introduction.

11. Charles Swindoll, *Come Before Winter and Share My Hope* (Portland, OR: Multnomah, 1985), 29.

Chapter 13—Rewriting the Past

1. The original source of this quotation is unknown.

2. Rick Warren, *The Purpose Driven Life: What on Earth Am I Here For?* (New York: HarperCollins, 2012), 32.

3. Ibid.

4. Dan Allender, *The Wounded Heart: Hope for Adult Victims of Childhood Sexual Abuse* (Colorado Springs, CO: NavPress, 1993), 30.

5. Alyce Faye Cleese and Brian Bares, *How to Manage Your Mother: Understanding the Most Difficult, Complicated and Fascinating Relationship in Your Life* (New York: HarperCollins, 2000), 8-9.

6. Lloyd John Ogilvie, *Lord of the Impossible* (Nashville: Abingdon Press, 1984), 129-30.

7. Aaron Fruh, *Bounce: Learning to Thrive Through Loss, Tragedy and Heartache* (Grand Rapids, MI: Baker Books, 2017), 126.

8. Robert S. McGee, *The Search for Significance,* rev. ed. (Nashville: W Publishing Group, 1998, 2003), 84-85.

9. John Ortberg, *Love Beyond Reason: Moving God from Your Head to Your Heart* (Grand Rapids, MI: Zondervan, 1998), 139.

10. David Seamands, *Healing Grace: Finding Freedom from the Performance Trap* (Colorado Springs, CO: Victor Books, 1988), 115.

11. McGee, *The Search for Significance,* 266.

12. Norman Vincent Peale, *Positive Imagine: The Powerful Way to Change Your Life* (New York: Ballantine Books, 1996), 17.

13. H. Norman Wright, *Self-Talk, Imagery, and Prayer in Counseling: A How-To Approach* (Dallas: Word Publishing, 1986), adapted, 186-96.

Chapter 14—Let the Spirit Lead You

1. John Ortberg, *The Me I Want to Be: Becoming God's Best Version of You* (Grand Rapids, MI: Zondervan, 2010), 97-98.

2. Charles R. Swindoll, *Living Above the Level of Mediocrity* (Dallas: Word, 1987), 94-95.

About the Author

H. Norman Wright, author of more than 90 books, is a well-respected Christian counselor who has helped thousands of people deal with grief, tragedy, and other concerns through books such as *When It Feels Like the Sky Is Falling* and *When the Past Won't Let You Go*. He also helps couples bring vibrancy to their relationships through seminars and his longtime bestsellers *Before You Say "I Do"* and *After You Say "I Do."* www.hnormanwright.com

I'll Never Forget That Day

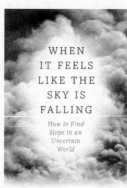

H. NORMAN WRIGHT

When It Feels Like the Sky Is Falling
by H. Norman Wright

The unexpected strikes each of us at some point in our lives. Those days when the sky feels as though it's closing in and our world is crumbling around us. A loved one dies... We survive a natural disaster... We witness a horrific event or act of terrorism. And we live in fear of what might happen as we step onto an airplane or watch as someone we love is admitted into the hospital.

How can we best respond to such shock and grief? Is it possible to feel safe again or to make sense of life in the aftermath?

Christian counselor H. Norman Wright has helped individuals cope in the wake of 9/11; Hurricane Katrina; the mass shootings at Aurora, Colorado and Las Vegas, Nevada; and other traumatic events. Here he offers compassionate guidance on facing—and growing from—the circumstances you fear most. You'll discover practical ways to prepare for the unexpected and find a path to real hope and peace—even in the midst of tragedy.

Is Your Yesterday Getting in the Way of Today and Tomorrow?

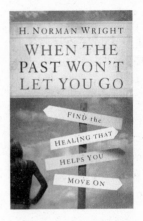

When the Past Won't Let You Go
by H. Norman Wright

Release your past to God once and for all with the help of respected Christian counselor H. Norman Wright, who has worked with grief-stricken individuals in the aftermath of 9/11, Hurricane Katrina, and mass shootings.

Whether you've experienced a major ordeal or a series of disappointments, it's impossible to move forward when painful emotions remain unaddressed and broken relationships stay unresolved. Reclaim hope for the future by...

- sorting through memories
- identifying lingering hurts
- overcoming former traumas
- grieving previous losses
- claiming forever freedom in Christ

Leave the past behind, experience fullness of life in the present, and look forward to the future. Healing awaits.

To learn more about Harvest House books and
to read sample chapters, visit our website:

www.harvesthousepublishers.com

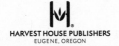

HARVEST HOUSE PUBLISHERS
EUGENE, OREGON